Praise for *A Doctor's Quest*

A Doctor's Quest offers a roller-coaster ride on a voyage into far-flung and sometimes dangerous territory, with thrills, spills, and occasional joy along the way. Read these stories of Gretchen Roedde's travel each year from small-town Ontario to the world's poorest countries in an effort to improve maternal health care, and marvel, admire, laugh, weep, and learn.

— Olive Senior, author of *Dancing Lessons, Working Miracles: Women's Lives in the English-Speaking Caribbean* and *Over the Roofs of the World*

This fine book demands, and deserves, slow and appreciative reading. Not only is it absorbing because it is beautifully written — Gretchen Roedde's voice is intimate and honest, allowing the reader to fully enter her experiences as a maternal health physician — it is also a deeply researched document providing anecdotal evidence of the real, terrifying inequities that still exist for women giving birth around the world.

— Isabel Huggan, author of *Belonging: Home Away from Home*

Gretchen Roedde tells a wrenching and powerful tale about how the wealthy and privileged on this planet are failing the weakest and the poorest, namely the women and girls around the world who perish, needlessly, while trying to give life. Her compassion, curiosity, and knowledge shine through in this fast-paced and no-holds-barred account of decades in the health-care trenches around the world, as do the resilience and strength of the women whose stories and voices Roedde brings us. Her deft touch and honesty transform deeply disturbing stories into a book that is also inspiring and full of hope.

— Joan Baxter, author of *Dust from Our Eyes: An Unblinkered Look at Africa*

I found *A Doctor's Quest* impossible to put down. It's full of vivid characters and situations, and at the same time is a breathtaking account of the lot of millions of impoverished women. This is a story we need to know, and Roedde, with her wide experience and no-nonsense compassion, is just the person to tell it.

— John Bemrose, author of *The Island Walkers*

Gretchen Roedde has braved civil war, government corruption, and her own self-doubt to prevent needless deaths of pregnant women and their babies. To read this impassioned, heart-wrenching book is to walk alongside a clear-eyed pathfinder who resists pat conclusions. I am inspired by her courage, challenged by her insights, and moved by her finely drawn portraits of women who are asking why they must risk death to give life.

— Rona Maynard, author of *My Mother's Daughter*

A wonderful read … a perspective that deserves and needs to be told, documenting the reflection and weaving the technical details in a cohesive manner.

— Dr. Michael Douglas, Healthinsights, Australia

A Doctor's Quest speaks in the voice of birthing women from the rural regions of fifteen of the poorest countries around the world. Their tales of bravery in the face of delivering without trained birth attendants and the joys and the complications that occur are the substance of the book. Weave in the public health perspective on interrelated themes of literacy, contraception, health care delivery, rural health work shortage, social disruptions, sexual violence, inefficient health care systems and corruption, and the book becomes a compelling treatise on maternal health.

— Dr. Peter Hutten-Czapski,
Canadian Journal of Rural Medicine

A Doctor's Quest

Second Edition

The Struggle for Mother-and-Child
Health Around the Globe

GRETCHEN ROEDDE

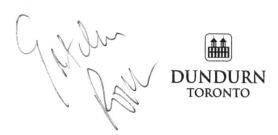

DUNDURN
TORONTO

Cover image: *Madonna and Child*, created and copyrighted by Linda Mustard and Gretchen Roedde.
Printer: Webcom, a division of Marquis Book Printing Inc.
Excerpt from Pablo Neruda's "Invisible Man" used with permission by the Fundación Pablo Neruda.

Library and Archives Canada Cataloguing in Publication

Roedde, Gretchen, author
   A doctor's quest : the struggle for mother-and-child health around
the globe / Gretchen Roedde. -- Second edition.

Includes bibliographical references and index.
Issued in print and electronic formats.
ISBN 978-1-4597-4332-8 (softcover).--ISBN 978-1-4597-4333-5 (PDF).--
ISBN 978-1-4597-4334-2 (EPUB)

   1. Maternal health services--Developing countries. 2. Maternal and
infant welfare--Developing countries. 3. HIV-positive persons--Care--
Developing countries. I. Title.

RG940.R64 2019   362.1982'0091724   C2018-906292-4
                                                  C2018-906293-2

1 2 3 4 5   23   22   21   20   19

 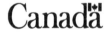 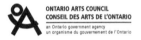

We acknowledge the support of the **Canada Council for the Arts**, which last year invested $153 million to bring the arts to Canadians throughout the country, and the **Ontario Arts Council** for our publishing program. We also acknowledge the financial support of the Government of Ontario, through the **Ontario Book Publishing Tax Credit** and **Ontario Creates**, and the **Government of Canada**.

Nous remercions le **Conseil des arts du Canada** de son soutien. L'an dernier, le Conseil a investi 153 millions de dollars pour mettre de l'art dans la vie des Canadiennes et des Canadiens de tout le pays.

Care has been taken to trace the ownership of copyright material used in this book. The author and the publisher welcome any information enabling them to rectify any references or credits in subsequent editions.
— *J. Kirk Howard, President*

The publisher is not responsible for websites or their content unless they are owned by the publisher.

Printed and bound in Canada.

VISIT US AT

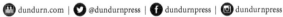 dundurn.com | @dundurnpress | dundurnpress | dundurnpress

Dundurn
3 Church Street, Suite 500
Toronto, Ontario, Canada
M5E 1M2

This book is in memory of Jens Hasfeldt. It commemorates our twenty-year friendship begun in Darfur, Sudan, in 1989 until Easter 2009, when he died of cancer. When he died, Jens was preparing a final mission to Papua New Guinea, a journey I continued in his stead.

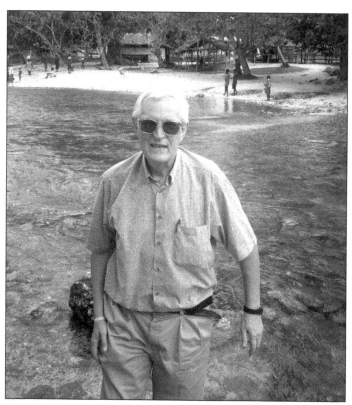

Jens Hasfeldt, Papua New Guinea, 2008.

CONTENTS

FOREWORD

The first two decades of the twenty-first century have shown unprecedented progress in the health of the people, that is, in improvements in the overall health of all of us in this globalized world. Hardly any village, even in the poorest and most remote corners of our ever smaller world, has not benefited from the positive effects of the health and medical revolution that humankind launched over the last century (think Ebola prevention and treatment advances, for example) and the practical results of which are now increasingly reaching all of us, from young to very old. In its wake "global health," as we now call it, has expanded exponentially, and every self-respecting country, university, or clinical constituency is somewhere involved in its exciting progress.

However, as with all rosy pictures, somewhere, to recall what Philip Roth said, there are human stains. In our case the stain concerns those who inevitably are being left behind, or who remain forgotten or somehow fail to attract attention to their piercing question — in whatever form — "Can my family or child please also …?" This is where our global health community has too many instances of a no-returning echo. Still, we are blessed to have Dr. Gretchen Roedde answer on our behalf.

Dr. Roedde and I met for the first time almost thirty years ago, either in Zambia or in Bangladesh — I think it may have been in Bangladesh. Later we discovered that we had a towering teacher in common: Dr. Rosemary McMahon of London and Liverpool, who, in the early days of international health, was the inspiration of many future global health leaders. When I met Gretchen Roedde, it was immediately clear to me that I had not a traditional Canadian physician in front of me but some kind of a global health warrior, someone who, without any respect for authority, would fiercely call to account the effectiveness of the big global health funders and implementing agencies, including those national and local health providers who would gladly play the global game, rather than prioritize the needs of their own poorest and most vulnerable. In the eyes of Dr. Roedde, money, effectiveness, and accountability are bureaucratic standards that remain meaningless unless they can be translated into the humaneness, caring, and empathy that the poorest, especially women and children, are often most in need of.

Many a warrior can be defeated or slain by the dragon: no such chance with Dr. Roedde, who takes on some of the darker forces of global health. She derives her staying power and influence from a rare combination of characteristics: unlike so many global health "advocates," she is not merely a talker; she is the real thing, one of those few global health leaders who actually practises medicine and health care, preventively, clinically, and epidemiologically — and everywhere in the world: in the remote and disadvantaged areas of the rich world (e.g., in her native Canada, with the isolated Ojibwe and Cree settlements) and all over the place in the most dangerous and far-flung villages in Africa, Asia, and the South Pacific. And then she translates those operational experiences with her patients into global health policy priorities, especially for the poorest mothers and children of this earth. She abhors bureaucracies but is nevertheless able to deal with them and often even convince them.

Dr. Roedde can communicate and write the most poignant stories about her work with gripping effect. Her recounts of her maternal and pediatric work read like the best adventure novels, with the difference that they are painfully true. You often feel as if you're there with her, with her struggle to find the best way to help the girl at risk of female genital mutilation, or to save the woman with a prolapse in the middle of the night in front of her hut somewhere, or the infant or child facing imminent death in the jungles of Africa, the Himalayan mountains, or some remote village in China or Ethiopia.

This book is a must-read for all global health professionals, be they of the older generations, millennials, or the even younger generations interested and motivated by today's global health challenges. Dr. Roedde should be congratulated on her ability to share with us her commitment to the weakest members of our global health community, a deeply personal commitment that has made such a difference in the lives of so many women and children around this world.

— Ok Pannenborg
October 2018

Ok Pannenborg was the World Bank's most senior technical health leader and director during the 1990s and 2000s, served as a director at the Pan American Health Organization (PAHO/WHO), was chairman of the Netherlands Government Commission on Global Health Research, and continues to chair various global health commissions and boards around the world.

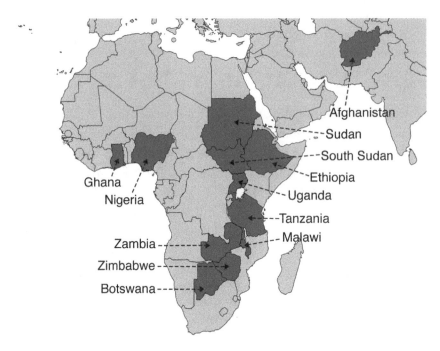

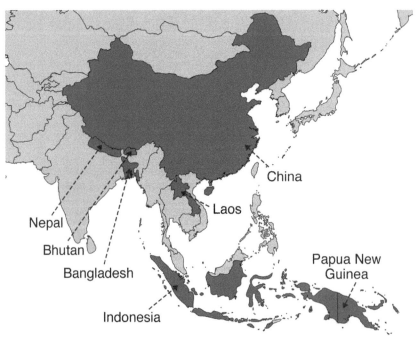

Introduction

Between 2000 and 2015, there were major achievements in reducing the deaths of pregnant women and children under five, with focused monitoring of specific goals and substantial increases in resource mobilization. Even though many countries did not meet the targets set for the 2015 Millennium Development Goals to improve maternal and child health, and the rate of change was uneven, momentum was established and lessons were learned to scale up existing and new interventions. Sub-Saharan Africa remains particularly challenged. The Countdown to 2030 adopted by the UN General Assembly in September 2015 addresses the broader Global Strategy for Women's, Children's and Adolescents' Health of Sustainable Development Goals.

Strengthened areas of attention include *nutrition; adolescent girls' reproductive health; quality of care; reproductive, maternal, and child health in conflict settings;* and *reducing inequity in access to health care within countries.*

Nutrition was one of the three pillars of Canadian support in the Muskoka Initiative; this important contribution is discussed later in this text. Fourteen countries globally have a prevalence of wasting (acute malnutrition greater than 10 percent), including fragile states such as South Sudan, also discussed in this edition. Even countries with improvements in maternal and child health showed persistent maternal anemia and stunting or chronic malnutrition of children under five, reflecting that underlying poverty and hunger are major determinants of health. If a pregnant woman is anemic, she is more likely to die if she has a post-partum hemorrhage, the leading cause of maternal deaths in poor countries. And malnutrition is a major determinant of deaths of children under five, contributing to 45 percent of those deaths. So the Countdown to 2030's focus on nutrition helps to address equity. Within countries, there are marked differentials in stunting between rich and poor quintiles. Stunting is chronic malnutrition, reflecting lack of food. Wealthy families have access to food even in times of scarcity such as famine, so the richest 20 percent of the population or quintile has low rates of stunting, unlike the poorest quintile for whom food security is challenged.

Adolescent girls' reproductive health is an extremely important focus. Teenaged pregnancy is high risk. Intergenerational sex is an important driver of the HIV epidemic (for example, the older married boyfriend who may have HIV and a school-aged girlfriend). Encouraging girls to remain in school is also linked to reducing maternal deaths and the deaths of children. Literate girls have lower rates of maternal death as well as of the deaths of their children under five. But girls are disadvantaged: in many countries, a pregnant school girl is expelled from school, while the father of the baby has no penalty. This is a factor in teenaged pregnant girls terminating pregnancy with unsafe abortion, leading to infection or death. In many countries, it is illegal for adolescent girls to access contraception without parental consent.

And yet, this was a missing piece in the Canadian Muskoka Initiative, reflecting the conservative policy agenda of the Harper government (2006–15). Family planning was barely supported, and there was no focus on adolescent girls.[1,2] Similarly, in the current (as of the time of writing) U.S. Trump Republican government, family planning support for developing country health services is now missing, even though this is the most cost-effective intervention to improve maternal and child health. So, while crucial, this area is very vulnerable to policy contexts of both developing countries (such as attacks on adolescent girls attending school in Nigeria) and donor countries (for example, the religious right as a base who oppose adolescent reproductive health) — even when the evidence shows that family planning reduces unsafe abortion, to which adolescents are particularly vulnerable.

Quality of care is highly variable, with poorer districts lacking staff, medicines, gloves, disinfectants, and water, which undermines improvement in health outcomes. In order to improve this, additional funding is required. In 2015, the Global Financing Facility was launched as the financing platform of the United Nations Secretary-General's Global Strategy for Women's, Children's and Adolescents' Health to promote universal coverage for, in particular, reproductive, maternal, newborn, child, and adolescent health.[3] Dr. Tim Evans at the World Bank was a major contributor to this policy.

Conflict settings are particularly challenging for the provision of reproductive, maternal, newborn, child, and adolescent health. Money is displaced from funding health to funding war. Members of military and peacekeeping organizations as well as non-governmental organizations (NGOs) have been implicated in sexual abuse of women and children and in the spread of HIV. The health system collapses, and distribution of food and medicines is disrupted. Women and children have to flee from their homes. But there are also opportunities for innovative solutions. Canada has helped fund NGOs doing integrated community case management of childhood illness in countries such as South Sudan, an important intervention for resource-poor settings, especially in conflict zones.[4]

Equity in access to health care within and between countries is still an elusive goal. Maternal mortality is nearly thirty times higher and child mortality fifteen times higher in poor countries than in high-income countries. The Global Financing Facility is in support of Every Woman Every Child. This movement is a strategy to accelerate international and national action and commitment by governments, UN agencies, civil society, and the private sector to place women, children and adolescents at the heart of development. It prioritizes investment in evidence-based high-impact strategies such as immunization, family planning, and nutrition, and scaling up additional supports in the continuum of care, with a transition to sustainable financing as countries become more developed and can better promote universal health coverage from domestic resources. This strategy was proposed by the World Bank to help close the $33 billion annual financing gap to meet the Sustainable Development Goals. Main contributors are the Norwegian, Canadian, American, and Japanese governments, the Bill and Melinda Gates Foundation, and Merck for Mothers.

Closing financial barriers still leaves cultural barriers. Maternal and neonatal health is culturally bound, since the customs of giving birth are specific to traditions. Health systems have trouble adapting our Western model to unique community-felt needs. Our challenge is to bring the skilled birth attendant as geographically and culturally close to the community as possible, as well as to make the costs of maternal health subsidized as a social good, rather than a system that requires a user to pay at the point of care. And we have to work with the complex dynamics that drive maternal health and maternal mortality.

Poverty drives maternal deaths. Maternal health is the most sensitive indicator of equity, and the most vulnerable to the loss of health workers through the brain drain to wealthier regions. We know that poor women are the most likely to die in pregnancy. They cannot access the care they need such as family planning, midwives to deliver their babies safely, or emergency obstetric care when things go wrong.

Gender inequality drives maternal deaths. Women with low status cannot negotiate with their families to part with their precious and limited income to pay for good care in labour and delivery. Young girls may be sold into marriage to pay off a family debt and become pregnant when they are too young for a safe delivery. Women with no power are subject to beatings, which increase in pregnancy, and in some countries, such as Bangladesh, can cause over 10 percent of maternal deaths. Canadian-funded research in Nigeria demonstrated that community-based interventions could raise awareness about intimate partner violence, which increases in pregnancy, and could help communities transform those patterns of behaviour.[5]

Child and maternal mortality are linked. Children's lives can be strengthened with interventions such as immunization, rehydration fluids for diarrhea, antibiotics for infection, treatment for malaria, and sleeping under insecticide-treated bed nets. More progress has been made in reducing the deaths of infants over one month and under five years than in improving neonatal and maternal health. Maternal and neonatal health requires an accessible health system that is integrated from the village level to small health centres with skilled birth attendants, and then up to the hospital level if emergency obstetric care is required. At the moment the staff are not there or the costs to access them are prohibitive. Currently, each mother in the developing world may lose one child to early death, and poor women are more likely to have a child die before his or her fifth birthday. In the fifty countries with the highest mortality rates, the average annual rate of decline in deaths of those under age five will need to almost double and in newborn deaths more than double to meet the 2015–30 targets. Eighty-one countries account for 95 percent of maternal deaths and 90 percent of children's deaths globally. These countries will need to be carefully tracked.

Female literacy improves maternal and child health. The girl who is not important enough to get an education is more likely to become pregnant early in adolescence, when she is more at risk of death from unsafe abortion or obstructed labour. She is less likely than her educated sisters to get the help she needs to bring children safely into the world. Girls with an education delay pregnancy and are better able to care for their children's illnesses. The educated and employed girl uses her money to pay for the family's food, health, and education. Female literacy is also closely linked with poverty — the poor are less likely to educate their girls, and the less literate are poorer than their educated counterparts.

The interventions to improve reproductive, maternal, newborn, child, and adolescent health are known. The essential interventions across the continuum of care — pre-pregnancy, pregnancy, birth, postnatal, infancy, childhood, and in the environment — are being carefully tracked as part of the Countdown to 2030. Tracking will not only address median coverage and the rate of change, but also what proportion of the gap is closed. A composite coverage index will also look at differences in coverage between the top and bottom income quintiles to assess equity. Similar tracking from 2000 to 2015 showed that under-five mortality from vaccine-preventable diseases such as measles declined the most, followed by pneumonia, diarrhea, and malaria with drops of more than 50 percent. Neonatal deaths fell less quickly, reflecting poor pregnancy care. Maternal deaths also have fallen less dramatically, with high rates of hemorrhage, hypertension, and sepsis. We know that delays in the family and among community healers who do not recognize there is a problem lessen the chances of successful delivery. Transportation difficulties such as lack of vehicles and often dangerous travel conditions cause delays in bringing labouring women to care and often make women feel that it is safer to deliver in their own communities. However, there should be no delays in getting pregnant women to proper facilities that provide prompt support and that have the necessary staff, equipment, drugs, and subsidized care.

We know we need to reduce these delays, but this requires subsidies and human and financial resources to be available to help communities understand warning signs. We also know that family planning, skilled birth attendants, and emergency obstetric care are needed, but religious, social, and financial barriers can hinder all of these.

There are complex links between infectious diseases such as HIV and malaria with maternal health. On the one hand, reducing HIV reduces maternal deaths, as some of these are linked to HIV. Similarly, reducing malaria improves maternal health as pregnant women are vulnerable to malaria. Between 2000 and 2015, coverage with intermittent preventive treatment for malaria for pregnant women increased from 3 to 11 percent. Pregnant women living with HIV who received anti-retrovirals increased from 1 percent to 66 percent. Diseases such as HIV and malaria have been highlighted on national and international agendas, and have mobilized money. Now a broader approach to catalyzing resources for reproductive, maternal, newborn, child, and adolescent health will help to close remaining gaps.

Global leadership for reproductive, maternal, newborn, child, and adolescent health is becoming stronger. Tracking policy changes is part of the Countdown to 2030: health service delivery inputs; legislative commitments such as maternity care and adolescent access to family planning; governance processes such as the presence of costed plans for maternal, newborn, and child health and maternal death audits; and financial investments from private and public sources.[6] Still, out-of-pocket expenses are more than 40 percent of total health expenditures in half of the Countdown countries, which will undermine access to skilled attendants at delivery and emergency obstetric care among other services.

In Papua New Guinea in 2009, I was working to address the issue of an apparent doubling of the deaths of pregnant women in the past decade, increases that took place despite a strong economy and massive foreign aid. There I met Theresa, a volunteer health worker struggling to understand why the women in her village continued to die. Her lament, tearfully shared with me in a clearing in the rain surrounded by hundreds of men, women, and children in her community, echoed my own understanding of the realities constraining women's lives:

> I am poor.
> I do not have the freedom that you have as a woman.
> One day my child was playing, the next day he had died.
> I have no education.
> Why are women dying giving life?
> I am tired of seeing HIV as the price of wealth.
> Where are our leaders? Why have they forgotten us?
> We are still waiting.

Combining Theresa's lament with my own lived experience and analysis, I have selected one-third of the countries in which I have worked with non-governmental agencies, governments, and the United Nations over more than three decades to reflect on my own doctor's quest to work in mother-and-child health, as a witness and technical adviser. This book is offered in the hope that collectively, we can put the last first and work to save the lives of women who consistently put themselves last in order to serve their children and communities.

Beginnings:

Haileybury, Ontario, Canada, 1987

In January 1987, the phone rang at four in the morning. I stumbled out of the bedroom to answer it, my heart beating rapidly. A crisp European voice asked, "Is Dr. Roedde there? The doctor who taught at the Liverpool School of Tropical Medicine in England last year? That's how I got your name."

The frantic pounding of my heart slowed. Thank God it wasn't an emergency.

"I'm calling from Geneva. Rosemary McMahon at Liverpool thought you might be interested in this job in Uganda. Could you be ready to go in two weeks?"

I was still struggling to wake up. "Yes, this is Dr. Roedde," I said sleepily. "Uganda?" I was dimly aware that in Uganda the civil war was just ending and the country was plagued by HIV/AIDS.

"It will be a tough assignment. I am Katja Janovsky. I've been working there for years with AMREF [African Medical Research Foundation] before coming to the World Health Organization [WHO]. Whole villages are dying of AIDS, thin, wasted people struggling to keep on living. But they're luckier than those who have died in the wars. There are fields that are still full of bones where Idi Amin has thrown the bodies of his enemies. I want you to be prepared."

I collected myself. I was awake now. Almost. With one hand on the phone, I stretched over to add grounds to the automatic coffee maker with the other and switched the pot on, trying to focus.

Katja explained. "I'm building a team for German Technical Assistance [GTZ, now GIZ]. We're going to help plan a primary health-care project in two poor, remote districts — Kabarole and Bundibugyo in western Uganda."

Even half asleep I knew that primary health care was the most basic level of health care and included immunization, mother-and-child health, nutrition, water and sanitation, and provision of essential drugs.

Katja continued. "GTZ wants to strengthen primary health care because it's low cost and saves the most lives. There will be a little hospital strengthening just to back up the primary level, but the major focus is to be on the poor. Can you go twice?"

As the caffeine hit my system, I learned that Katja wanted me for two missions: first, for this German project that she would be coordinating, and then for an AMREF mission that I would conduct on my own.

Over our clear transatlantic line, Katja explained more about the assignments. "There will be a couple of months for you to go home between the two missions, each of which will be four weeks long. The AMREF job is to strengthen the training for several different cadres of primary health staff, work you've already been doing in Liverpool. I know you've worked in Canada's own developing world training Indigenous health workers and have had students from Africa, Asia, and the South Pacific at Liverpool. But isn't it time you take this opportunity to work in the same conditions as your Liverpool students?"

Eager, I answered, "Yes," but I tried not to let my nervousness show in my voice. "Katja, these will be my first assignments in Africa."

After I got off the phone and while my family continued to sleep, I wondered how I would actually undertake these challenging journeys and how I could juggle them with the responsibilities I had to my family and my northern Ontario patients where I served as a locum physician in the small towns of Haileybury, New Liskeard, Latchford, Cobalt, and Temagami. At the same time I tried to pull together the fragments I knew about

Uganda, many learned from my father, a retired librarian who is currently an artist, or from my husband, Jim, a historian who could provide political commentary on probably every country in the world over his gourmet-cooked meals.

A week later, with a cursory knowledge of German and the aid of a dictionary, I picked my way through the German contract that had arrived by courier. It was a delicate and difficult task, but by then I was fully engaged and energized at the prospect of going to Africa, something I had long wanted to do. But my excitement didn't dispel my anguish at leaving my family for so long. When my daughter, Anna, was nineteen months old, I had left her for three months to study in Liverpool. I cried every day and was devastated when I returned and discovered that she didn't recognize me. Over the years, I knew my children, Anna and Alec, who were then respectively eight and five years old, had become used to parents with alternating travel schedules. After Alec was born, it was my turn to hold down the fort while Jim, who worked as an Indigenous land claims historian and travelled extensively to Indigenous communities throughout North America, moved to Toronto for several months for a Supreme Court land claim trial. And so, with Jim's encouragement and reassurance that he could handle my absence by rearranging his schedule to work from home, and after a discussion with my children that Mum would be away for a little while, I knew I could go.

What I didn't know was that answering Katja's phone call that early morning would change the way I worked for the rest of my life.

> Give me for my life all lives,
> give me all of the suffering of the whole world.
> I am going to turn it into hope.
> Give me all the joys,
> even the most secret
> because otherwise how will these things be known?
> I have to tell them. Give me the labours of every day,
> for that's what I sing.
> — Pablo Neruda, "The Invisible Man"

1

I Am Poor:

Uganda, Sudan, and South Sudan

First Mission, Uganda, 1987

We lurched along the rutted red *murram* (earth) road, the dark forest gleaming green and black against the violet sky. Huge flowering trees dropped flamboyant, jacaranda, and bougainvillea blossoms, delighting me with the feel of their feather-light lavender, fuchsia, and orange petals. The noisy chatter of monkeys in the low branches of the trees melded with the calls of mysterious new birds and the strange grunts from animals I could only imagine on my first time in a jungle. When four-foot Twa pygmies ran to meet us, smoking strange pipes and offering monkey-furred objects for sale, the sight of them was straight out of a storybook. The magical quality of the moment seemed to belie the challenge of this journey.

Our young university-educated driver, Paul Mpanga, had spent hours waiting in long queues at various filling stations so we would have enough fuel for the several-day trip to the west and back. Once we were on our way with jerry cans precariously loaded on the roof, he joked, "In Uganda you can tell a drunk driver because he drives in a straight line instead of

swerving to avoid potholes." Many times we got stuck in the wet mud and had to get out and push the Jeep.

We were travelling to the west, several hours from the chaos of Kampala, Uganda's capital. Our work was to assess the staff and supply needs in health facilities, from small rural clinics to hospitals in these isolated rural regions. The health workers — all of them unpaid — did what they could in these most difficult circumstances. But the only foods, harvested from the local *shamba* (family farm), were a few bananas and plantains. They were a major food source at all times, but especially in this period of war and poverty when no one could afford chicken, eggs, fish, or goat. This lack of nutrients resulted in the starving children we would see on the wards, with their grossly swollen bellies and thin, wasted arms.

I had never seen such suffering, had never fully understood that the photographs and newscasts of famine and HIV victims were of such terribly real human beings. In the first hospital, on our first day, I had to struggle with nausea and keep my face tight with control, since I felt I was shattering into small pieces. I glanced at my companions, who seemed unmoved or perfectly able to cope, and became painfully aware of my inexperience. But how could one possibly get used to this?

In the crowded outpatient department, patients in ragged clothing spilled in from the veranda, and naked children and babies cried. Mothers seemed listless and resigned. The smell of urine permeated the room. Nurses used the same needle to inject many different people, wiping the needle on their worn dresses between patients. One nurse, named Beatrice, asked me plaintively, "What else can we do? We know how bad things are here, we know we are spreading infection, but there are no supplies, and even the water we use isn't clean."

These hospitals in the centre of the AIDS epidemic had no gloves for health workers, no condoms, and few needles. We shuddered, remembering the well-stocked warehouses we had left behind days earlier in the capital, where our fellow jet-set development health personnel were busy joining one another at the Entebbe Sailing Club on Lake Victoria for drinks and sailing, making dates for tennis, and hiring better cooks and houseboys.

In a hospital in Fort Portal, on the pediatric ward, we saw three small children who were so pale they appeared to be white, not black. They were

severely anemic, suffering from malaria, and in desperate need of blood transfusions. The families were being shouted at by the nurses, who were demanding money that the families didn't have. Two children were turned away. One small girl, Flavia, appeared to be about four years old and was a little better dressed than the two left to die. Since there was no blood bank, once her mother was able to get enough paper Uganda shillings from the other members of the family to pay for treatment, the mother herself was strapped up to donate blood. This direct transfusion, from mother to child, was done without her being tested for HIV. There were no test kits.

I knew the facts and had read the reports. More than one in six children would die before they were five. Each mother could lose one child. The poor, because they can't afford enough food, have higher death rates for their children. So children who die from infection are usually malnourished. But nothing had prepared me for this reality.

On the wards the listless, wasted sick crowded together, lying side by side on the floor. Many of them were children, with swollen bellies, loose, dehydrated skin, and unresponsive eyes. They were dying from diarrhea, measles, malaria, malnutrition, and AIDS. I had never seen so many people near death in one place, many with illnesses that could be inexpensively prevented and treated. One mother, Ruth, looked into my eyes with beseeching intensity. She tried to coax drops of water from a dirty rag into her baby's dry mouth, and then tried again without success to squeeze milk from her own thin breasts. Without milk, with only filthy water, this baby would die. I looked around the ward. Ruth was one of many. Huddled on the floor, about twenty mothers all attempted to feed their starving, dehydrated babies — children who were too weak even to cry with hunger. I struggled not to weep, myself, as we made rounds through the wards. How could this be happening? How could there be so little help?

But we, too, came close to not being here to help.

———

After a seven-hour drive to Toronto, a long transatlantic flight to London, another ten hours to Nairobi, and a hop to Entebbe, I arrived in Uganda just before dusk. I was disoriented and exhausted but exhilarated. I had

expected to be met, but no one raised a sign with my name and no one was searching for a Canadian doctor. I needed to find my way to the German Embassy in Kampala, almost an hour's drive away, but had no idea where the embassy was and knew at this hour that it would be closed.

Surveying the boisterous sea of Ugandan taxi drivers aggressively offering their services, I struggled to stay calm and eventually chose a driver who seemed the least threatening, a slight man who had a soft smile and a gentle face. He ushered me into a beat-up cab, and we drove off toward Kampala. After passing through several army checkpoints "manned" by boy soldiers, he deposited me at a "major" hotel. Four stars adorned its shabby entrance, and a few other expatriate customers wandered the lobby. In my room I could hear the sound of sporadic gunfire in the streets, making me realize that the civil war hadn't really ended.

When I finally met up with Katja the following morning at a white-washed Entebbe guest house where she was staying, she informed me that our mission was in jeopardy. The German government was trying to cancel the project because of the current political instability. We now needed to convince them otherwise.

I cringed inwardly. The gunfire had frightened me into weeping and praying the night before, so I found no encouragement in the fact that the Germans had withdrawn support for our work and intended to cancel our mission because it was considered too dangerous.

Katja assembled everyone to plan a strategy for our meeting with the German Embassy. In Uganda for a month on another assignment for the World Bank, she had travelled upcountry already and thought the Germans were overreacting. David Porter, a Scot who had been working with her in the inland area, agreed. He seemed fearless and had extensive experience in harsh developing countries. Friedrich and Gerhardt, both Germans, completed the team. Their job as architect-builders was to plan any physical rehabilitation of the clinics and hospitals we would support.

At the embassy we met with the German chargé d'affaires. Katja took command. Softening her forceful personality with a flirtatious smile, she insisted they permit us to go ahead, since we were already here. She asserted that if the German Embassy was too frightened to let the two German nationals help, we — an Austrian, a Canadian, and a Scot — would go on

our own. The embassy conceded, somewhat horrified that two women and a short Scot were contemplating travel without the two obviously more capable Germans to accompany us.

In charge of the Fort Portal hospital in the poor district of Kabarole was Dr. Ingrid, a German surgeon well loved by Yoweri Kaguta Museveni's army. President Museveni had come to power after fighting a civil war in the bush using thousands of soldiers, many of them small boys.[1] Dr. Ingrid had worked tirelessly behind the lines in the war and had lost her African husband to other women somewhere along the way. She was truly a formidable presence with her blond hair back-combed high in a beehive and her polished white shoes click-clacking over feces-stained floors.

Dr. Ingrid's first priority for improved health care, she told us in no uncertain terms, was to obtain German funding for a neurosurgical ward. She had been treating soldiers with gunshot wounds and head injuries. Most of these men had died from post-operative infections, since they had to be nursed together with infectious cases on the crowded wards. We suggested, to Dr. Ingrid's disgruntlement, that rainwater tanks on the roof might be more important for a hospital lacking in basic cleanliness. And a clean operating room that could provide Caesarean sections for obstructed labour would save the lives of pregnant women as well as those of soldiers.

David Porter was so angry he almost shouted, "You have no clean water! This is a filthy hospital and you can't make your patients better in a place like this. You have to start with the basics."

Friedrich, Gerhardt, Katja, and Dr. Ingrid took themselves off to a corner to continue the discussion in German. I caught a phrase or two and knew our team was attempting to placate the surgeon by explaining our priorities and reconciling them with her own.

David and I stood outside for a few minutes in the sunlight as I tried to regain my composure. He could tell I was having a hard time. I was a neophyte, stunned by what I was seeing and trying to stand firmly on the shifting ground of my own preconceptions of what this trip would be like. He smiled. "I've just what you need, lass. I'm afraid it isn't a wee dram of a good single malt whisky, but I'll give you a good slug of *waragi* [local rum] when we get back to the guest house. That will give you some perspective."

As we accompanied Dr. Ingrid through the rest of the hospital, I clenched my jaw so I wouldn't cry. What could I do for this emaciated young man who weighed just over ninety pounds? He was dying of tuberculosis and AIDS, and coughed quietly as he gazed at me helplessly with enormous dark eyes in a bony face that would soon be just a skull. Never had I imagined there could be so little help for such overwhelming problems, so much slow death among children and their parents. At night, back at the guest house room with its cracked and peeling floorboards and broken windows, with a bucket of water in which floated bits of bark and debris for my own basic needs, I gave in and sobbed. I held my fist against my teeth to keep from wailing, knowing my colleagues were in rooms near mine, only thin walls separating us.

For days, then weeks, we visited all the health facilities in Kabarole and Bundibugyo, two impoverished regions in western Uganda. David Porter, with his irreproducible Scottish accent, pointedly summed up the extreme challenges of the situation that confronted us daily. "That last trip I took out to that remote health centre to see what they needed was tough. Army deserters were still floating about. I was on an isolated road between villages. When we responded to the shouts we heard in the distance, we initially sped up to see what was going on. But we quickly turned around. There was a guy in a tree being lynched by shouting armed men."

Friedrich and Gerhardt planned the physical rehabilitation of the facilities, rebuilding necessary in this impoverished area of post-conflict Uganda. They strutted importantly around, muttering in German with tape measures. Katja and I collaborated with the hospital superintendents and the midwifery school principals to outline improved in-service training for the health workers. Training had been hospital-based, but to serve the poor who lived in the rural areas, a stronger community-based approach was needed. At a local Catholic nursing school we suggested they provide midwifery training to better prepare staff to help pregnant women, since the poor usually delivered at home with an untrained birth attendant, and described how Germany could organize and fund the project.

I found Katja quite intimidating. She deftly took control, she was confrontational, and she was completely committed. I was hesitant to confide in her about how overwhelmed I sometimes felt by everything I

was learning and seeing. She piled on the work, and I was sleeping only an hour or two a night. How could I ever meet her expectations? She was impatient with my inexperience, so I tried to stay out of her way. At one point she brought out her Swiss army knife. "Do you want to see how this works?"

I was curious and moved closer. She opened it up to the tweezers. "Like this," she said, pulling hairs painfully out of my arm. I grimaced uneasily.

By the end of the mission, we had a sense of measured optimism, knowing those facilities were going to receive help. There would be no neurosurgical ward, but we had plans for rainwater tanks, medical equipment, and training for skilled birth attendants and others providing basic health care for the poor. It would be too late for Ruth and her baby, but hopefully other mothers wouldn't have to suffer the way she had.[2]

SECOND MISSION, UGANDA, 1987

The second project took me to the town of Mbale, northeast of Kampala, to assess training schools for health workers and suggest changes in the curriculum and teaching methods to make them more relevant for poor mothers and children. This would involve a shift in thinking and training with more hands-on work at the community level in fundamental primary health care.

When I arrived in Mbale, the woman in charge of Canadian support for the medical assistant training school welcomed me with an offer of a hot eucalyptus-scented bubble bath. It was far more lavish than the treatment received by the Ugandan students who had arrived just before I did, escorted by the army from their previous school in the town of Gulu in northern Uganda through many miles of active fighting.

I talked to a young man named Joseph who told me, "In the morning in front of the training school we would count the dead. How many were they? Had the women been raped? Did we know them?"

Another bright student, Christopher, had diagonal tribal markings on his face. "Our lives have been saved by the army that escorted us to safety. We are so grateful to be studying, even if we have no teachers. How could our professors keep coming to work? They are too poor and have to earn a living somehow. We know the government has no money for their salaries."

Doubled up in the dormitory with the students from Mbale, the newly arrived students studied and copied one another's notes with broken pencils on loose sheets of paper. The school principal had stolen all the beds to give to his own extended family, which had been displaced by the northern war, so these students were left with neither beds nor blankets and little food.

I travelled farther to visit training schools for nurses, midwives, pharmacists, and lab technicians, and then returned to Fort Portal in the Kabarole district in western Uganda to see the medical assistant training school. Like the school in Mbale and all the other places I had evaluated, it had no supplies and its students were hungry with their allotment of one bowl of porridge per day.

The hospital in Fort Portal was no longer overwhelming. As I toured Dr. Ingrid's hospital with the medical assistant students, the smell of shit now seemed normal. My hands hung loose at my sides; I no longer had them clenched in my pockets. I watched the students, glad they would be learning how to care for the sick and sad patients, to care for pregnant and delivering women, and believed we were building something stronger and better.

The students, however, were still hospital-based. Due to the ongoing instability in the area, they were unable to visit the remote rural health centres where they could learn practical skills. They couldn't get enough experience delivering babies. Poor women couldn't afford a hospital-based midwife and had to deliver at home.

It took fifteen years to establish clinical training for midwives, and as a result of that developmental work I was able to watch Hannah, a clinical

tutor, demonstrate how to operate the vacuum to help pull a baby out. The poor mother who previously could only afford to deliver at home had been able to reach a subsidized health centre that had midwives. But she had grown too tired to push. The cervix was fully dilated and the head was there, but the baby had started to show signs of distress. Hannah had observed this, listening to the late slowing of the fetal heart after the mother's contractions. Three uniformed students stood proudly with the midwife, one holding a blanket to carry the baby over to the warm table to be checked, one keeping the vacuum extractor working, and one passing instruments to the midwife.

By 2002, training schools for health workers were also implementing many of the recommendations we had made more than a decade earlier. Much higher numbers of nurse-midwives were now trained at mission facilities, which went a long way to improve the numbers of deliveries of poor women conducted by skilled birth attendants. Project funding from different development partners was channelled through one main implementing organization — in this case still AMREF but no longer with separate projects from different donors. The Fort Portal hospital, too, had been upgraded with the money from GTZ. Poor patients were still crowded on the wards, but the air of desperation had diminished. A more buoyant busyness emanated from the staff. The project we had helped establish in Fort Portal and Bundibugyo would later be cited as a best case practice in the fight against HIV.

In 1987, though, all of those advances remained a dream. The violence continued to put me on edge. One student, Victoria, had been shot. When I met with her peers, they described what a good student she had been. She was now paralyzed and in a wheelchair, her career over. I felt powerless. Improving the curriculum wouldn't help Victoria. How could I make the world any safer for these fine young people who wanted so much to acquire skills to help their poor communities?

We continued to visit dim, unlit health centres in a secure area where the students learned from experienced graduates. I noted that "assault" was a common diagnosis. Women, especially when they were pregnant, routinely faced beatings from their husbands or were slashed by their spouses with *pangas* (machete-like blades).

One nurse in an outpatient clinic tended to a pregnant woman named Maria, who had huge bruises and gashes on her slim body after being assaulted by her husband. The nurse showed two students how to treat her with injectable penicillin. In fact, she treated everything — malaria, pneumonia, body pains — with penicillin. I cringed. She even explained that when the penicillin — the good medicine — ran out, it would be replaced by whatever was available until that ran out. I wasn't sure what to do. Should I openly disagree with her?

Maybe she knew better. Perhaps the patients used any pretext to get antibiotics. They could give them at home later if a child got pneumonia. Because while waiting for another pre-packed kit of drugs that would take five or six weeks to arrive from Denmark, patients would stop coming and women would cease bringing their sick children. The risk of being raped several times by soldiers on patrol along the way to the health centre was simply not worth it if there were no medicines. The fear of rape was another reason pregnant women didn't come to a health centre for care.

Nevertheless, poor women were discovering how to care for their sick children and were being taught how to read. They learned how to recognize warning signs in labour and delivery when they helped one another give birth. These women always greeted us with dancing. In spite of insurmountable losses and poverty, joy was alive.

Two women invited me into their dance, laughing, swaying side to side, hips close as the eyes of the men and women in the village lit up. The women drew me closer with a bright piece of multi-coloured fabric, the three of us connected by the cloth, our bodies moving together. "Ulululu," sang the audience, the rejoicing sound of tongue giving praise. Our bare feet stamped on the dirt, and four small children rushed to join us, their waists twisting in a sensuous rhythm, grinning wildly. I wanted to understand this, to learn that I, too, could be grateful for this day and for their greeting.

———

As I travelled upcountry visiting training schools, I felt more confident. I was less frightened of the army checkpoints and soldiers. Fortified by the Gravol I took for motion sickness and the nausea from recurring migraines, I was relaxed. I managed to get through all the army checkpoints without becoming too wound up. At one point, a shabbily clad soldier, who couldn't have been older than twelve or thirteen, peremptorily told me I needed an official permit. He gave me a small piece of paper with a rubber-stamped drawing of a blue pussycat. I held it with slightly trembling hands until the next checkpoint, where I traded it for a pink pig. These child soldiers fighting a civil war were controlling traffic with animal stamps.

SPIRIT
I'm asked if it's good
To be back in the land
Of the living. I say
I left it.

My spirit left behind
with eye-sunken children
ribs poking through
bellies swollen.

My spirit left behind
with handless arms outstretched
grasping for coins
ever hopeful.

My spirit ever soaring
to lush hills on borders
past fields full of bones
thrown by monsters.

Somewhere it's lost, caught in
trucks full of schoolgirls
singing and
swaying to music.

Past soldiers at checkpoints,
storefronts where tailors'
feet pounding treadles
keep life moving.

Near mothers clothed with colour,
water on head,
child on back nursing life
from so little.

My spirit left behind
in orphans' sweet smiles
hands touching our hair
hugging closely.

My spirit ever soaring,
grunt of hippo in garden,
night drumming, sacred ibis
bird wings flashing.

Loss striking everyone,
beautiful suffering
moves me and moves me
and moves me.

I'm asked if it's good
to be back in the land
of the living. I say
I left it.

— Gretchen Roedde, Uganda, 1987

SUDAN, 1989

I returned home a different woman. I didn't know then that the work I had done in Uganda would ultimately lead to such positive changes. I sat off by myself, awkward and sad, haunted by Ugandan ghosts. I thought of the American Catholic priest, Father John, who had been in Fort Portal for less than a year. When we met him, he apologized for not having done much in the year that he had been there. He was worried he had only been able to teach the unemployed youth to repair vehicles and to work planting gardens, growing castor plants whose oil he used for everything from motor oil to caring for patients in the hospital. Father John had also created an electrification system for the Catholic hospital and surrounding community. Would I ever accomplish that much? Africa had called me into its heart.

Two years after my trips to Uganda, I found myself back in Africa. Katja had invited me to participate in another GTZ primary health-care project to visit and assess government health facilities and midwifery schools in Sudan.

I soon discovered that one of the biggest challenges to maternal health in many parts of Africa, Sudan without exception, is the damage caused by female genital mutilation (FGM), or circumcision.

Dr. Mohammed Hassan Saeid, one of our accompanying Sudanese counterparts, constantly talked to hospital staff and students about the dangers of female circumcision in each school. He warned that it was against the Koran to defile the body and that it was forbidden by law.

Dating back to Pharaonic times, though illegal in Sudan, FGM is widely practised. Most midwives perform it for a small fee. At a minimum, the tip of the clitoris is removed. More often the entire clitoris is resected so there can be no female sexual pleasure. Sometimes the labia minora and majora are also cut off with a surgical knife for the wealthy, or with an unclean instrument for the poor, who can easily die of infections as a result. Poor women are already at higher risk of dying in labour, since they can't afford to be delivered by a midwife or have emergency obstetric care when things go wrong.[3] Poor women with FGM are more likely to tear and experience other obstetric complications. And poor women are more likely to give birth when they are still young adolescents, making their deliveries already high risk.

Often it is the mothers who take their young daughters to be circumcised so they will be "clean" for their future husbands. Even women whose husbands are educated and don't support female genital mutilation will sneak their small daughters away to be circumcised. It is so much easier to blame men. But the uncomfortable truth is that too frequently it is women who behave in oppressive ways to one another. The oppressed become the agents of their own social control. It is more complex than women's economic dependence on men in most of the world.

We were horrified by the screams of pregnant women on the delivery wards whose labours were much more difficult after genital mutilation. Others suffered fistulas that leaked urine after delivery. Fistulas are abnormal passages between organs such as the bladder, vagina, and rectum, and can lead to life-threatening infections. The constant leakage of bodily fluids also causes these women to be excluded socially, unable to participate in religious, family, and community events. Many of these women with fistulas are automatically divorced by their husbands and have no means of economic support.

One midwife, Yasmin, reminded us that these women were lucky. They hadn't died of infection as small girls.

That was my first direct encounter with FGM. Yasmin showed me the models she used to teach delivery: they had to be specially adapted from rubber tires to show a birth passage with no external genitalia, since these were totally removed in most of the women she delivered.

She continued softly. "After delivery, women are sewn up, allowing just a small passage for urine and menses to flow. After the birth, her spouse will seek other partners while she breastfeeds. When he wishes her to conceive again, perhaps in two years, it might require his knife to make it possible for her to have sex with him again."

Progress against FGM is slow. Many challenges that could be more easily solved have been addressed with ineffective "solutions." Poor children are more likely to suffer from malnutrition. Our joint Sudanese and expatriate team discovered that UNICEF had trained nurses on methods of growth monitoring to detect malnutrition, which is more pronounced in girls, who are less often brought to clinics and are given less food at home. But none of the facilities used the monitoring. Either weighing scales were lacking or there were no "road to health" cards on which to record weight. Furthermore, the available cards had been printed backward, possibly by a Westerner unsure about the direction of Arabic script. This in turn confused health workers. How to plot the growth — right or left? And so this vital record had been omitted from the child welfare check.[4]

Leaving the ice and snow-covered lake of my northern Ontario town at the end of January for Africa had sounded like a challenging change. But now I needed time to think. The relentless pace of our visits to health facilities and NGOs had given me no chance to reflect.

The dazzling bright sunny days that mysteriously shifted into nights where the temperature suddenly dropped disoriented me. When a political coup threatened, my colleagues and I got a chance to slow down. Because curfews confined us to our guest house while the army patrolled, we sat in the courtyard and watched the vast purple fade to a black star-filled sky. Over furtively drunk whisky, we talked about the soldiers and their guns, trying to absorb our shock and fear in this dangerous, vulnerable world. Our anguish seeped out into the night.

Before I left Canada it had taken me two weeks to convince the Sudanese ambassador in Toronto to grant me a visa because of a general strike and the lack of security. With the fighting in the south of Sudan between the northern Arab Muslims and the southern animist Christians, the political situation was highly unstable. The pervasiveness of political chaos that plagued so much of the continent was becoming a stark reality for me. The ongoing violence and civil war had depleted government coffers in Sudan, worsening poverty in many regions. After another week, though, I finally arrived, disoriented, in Khartoum.

I was delighted to see David Porter, who would again handle the medical equipment assessment, and met the other team members: Klaus, the German team leader, an expert in managing essential drug supplies; Jens Hasfeldt, a pharmaceutical specialist from Denmark who would determine how to manage the project; Rumishael Shoo, a Tanzanian public health doctor; and three Sudanese counterparts, all high-ranking male officials in the health sector, who carried with them voluminous briefing reports about the health situation in the country and would act as translators. After a day of meetings and preparation, we set off for northern Sudan.

Our small low-flying plane swooped along the ground close enough to see oceans of sand, camels driven by brightly clad tribesmen, great villages of tents springing out of nowhere, and women wearing loose, vibrant clothing carrying babies on their backs. Grey-green shadows lined the almost empty riverbeds where the moist earth allowed short grasses to grow. But as you gazed past the riverbeds, the colour changed to the dark yellow of Saharan sand. The choppy ride was familiar to me from years of travelling by bush plane in northern Ontario to isolated Ojibwe and Cree settlements.

After a short two-day stay in the wealthy Red Sea Hills and Northern Provinces where German development aid was certainly not needed, we set out for Darfur. Fifteen years later this region was to become notoriously familiar to Westerners. The government of Sudan refused to take humanitarian action in the wake of outright genocide and denied the occurrence of the slaughter of hundreds of thousands of people, killing witnesses and destroying mass graves.

In Darfur we planned to link up with NGOs in several areas to assess the health-care needs of both the internally displaced people from the south (animist Christians) and the residents of this deprived region. Our Muslim Sudanese colleagues, led by Dr. Saeid, wanted to limit our knowledge of the war in the south and forbade us from interacting with these NGOs and hearing their stories. "Do not see them, and if you do see them, do not believe what they tell you. They are interfering in politics, which are none of their business, and they will never understand." The war in the south was less a religious war than a fight over resources. The country's political strife was restraining humanitarian aid — GTZ had closed a project in the south due to the fighting, and the Muslim northern government in Khartoum was reluctant to allow any support to go to the hated southerners.

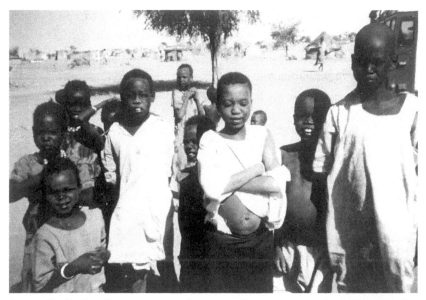

Internally displaced young men gather at a refugee camp run by MSF in Darfur, Sudan.

The many people fleeing the war had added to the burden on the health services in Darfur, and we hoped we could strengthen health services here. But we didn't understand the depth of the cultural hatred between these groups, fuelled by the competition for food in the context of drought, as well as for control over the oil and gold in the south. Out of the prying eyes of our Sudanese colleagues, we managed to visit a refugee camp run by Médecins Sans Frontières (MSF).

We met Birgit, a Belgian nurse-midwife who looked after the pregnant women, treated their malaria, and delivered their babies in the camps, working with few supplies. Her face was lined and exhausted. She was frustrated at government indifference and the lack of progress.[5] "Anger is so deep here," she told us wearily. "A few months ago, trainloads of hundreds of southerners were sent by rail to safety in Darfur. But the local people didn't want them. The trains were set on fire by the locals, and all the southerners were killed." So we worried that the Sudanese government would resist German aid coming into an area that would serve these unwanted refugees from the south.

Birgit explained. "Death rates are increased in these camps if people from different villages are thrown together. If we keep village and cultural structure as intact as possible, it improves the health of individuals, especially the more vulnerable women and children. So in forming these camps, MSF places people from the same or adjacent villages together so that these community bonds can help people find their new place and rebuild more quickly."

We were glad we had disobeyed our Sudanese hosts to visit the MSF camp. But we paid a price when the army shot at our retreating vehicle because Klaus had been unable to produce an official travel permit for our forbidden visit. The north-south conflict, or the poverty, or the internally displaced refugees, however, couldn't be held responsible for all of Darfur's woes. The clinic and hospital drugstores were full of unusable supplies, none of which could be removed. New supplies sat on the porch outside, spoiling in the heat.

On one inspection, Jens and Huda, a new Sudanese team member who was a pharmacist, found yard-high piles of medicines that were years past their expiry date. There were heaps of used needles and syringes and spoiled packages of oral rehydration salts. Frustratingly, we discovered this had nothing to do with the political situation but was due to complex bureaucratic ineffectiveness. None of the medicines could be disposed of until a particular committee had been formed, and such a committee was administratively impossible because of insurmountable red tape in the health facility.

The team planned to travel to a remote village several hours' drive across the Sahara. Our MSF friends advised us to bring sleeping bags, water, food, and flashlights to this severely deprived area. Nonsense, Klaus, our team leader, told us. "It's all been arranged," he said. Klaus had sent a message to an agricultural project also funded by Germany in the village of Kutum we were to visit. He told us provisions would be waiting for us. Reluctantly, we agreed, but to be on the safe side I brought one sleeping bag, juice, water, granola bars, dried soup, and a few other items.

We set off in the shimmering heat. The glare stung our eyes. Our Jeep lurched across the deeply furrowed desert. We saw white-robed, turbaned men in a *souk* (open market) selling piles of yellow, green, brown, and red grains and spices. The iridescent lake on the horizon kept receding as we got closer and was eventually revealed to be an ocean of sand. We wondered how our driver could find his way with no markings, no road, and just faded criss-crossing Jeep tracks from the travellers who had preceded us. At dusk we arrived in Kutum. Our Sudanese colleagues bickered with Klaus over the size of their per diems. They held him responsible, which wasn't fair, since the rates were set by GTZ, not by him.

With tight, angry lips, Klaus knocked on the door of a largely empty house, the base of another GTZ project where we were to sleep. The door was answered by a tall, clean-shaven German agriculturalist. While he was annoyed at our arrival on his doorstep, he was astonished that we expected him to feed and accommodate us. He hadn't been informed that we were coming. There were no beds, no bedding, and no stores of food in this lavish house. "This was built for me two years ago. I'm an agricultural adviser. But now I'm packing to go home. The project has been cancelled. I haven't been able to do any work here. The rate of rainfall is decreasing so fast that no one, not even Germans, will be able to improve production." Klaus seemed sheepish. The mood of the team was definitely deteriorating. We were tired from the long drive and furious with ourselves that we hadn't listened to our contacts in MSF.

Huda had trained in the United Kingdom. In Sudan she had never travelled outside Khartoum. She wrinkled her brow with distaste and peered doubtfully down at her patent leather high-heeled shoes. With flashlights in hand, our mixed team of formally dressed Sudanese and safari-clad expatriates carefully inched along the darkened village paths, searching for a place that could sell us food.

It was late, nearly midnight, when we returned to the GTZ project house. We gave all the bedding we could scrounge to our Sudanese colleagues, who were still threatening to strike over the size of their per diems. I had saved one slim blue rolled-up piece of foam for me to sleep on. As the night deepened, I started to shiver. My teeth chattered as the temperature dropped, so I reached over to my bag to grope for more clothing, finding a thin sweater, a pair of pants, a long-sleeved blouse, and another scarf. Fumbling in the dark, I piled these over (sweater, blouse, scarf) and under (trousers) my dress.

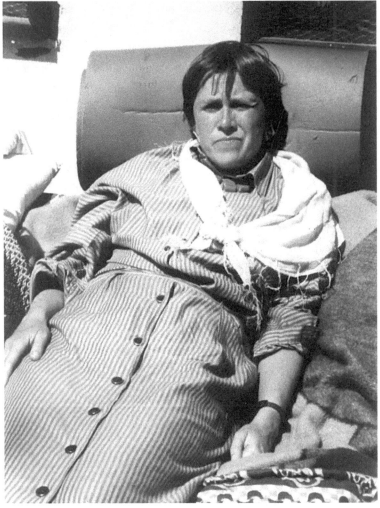

The author settled down to sleep in Darfur, Sudan.

The next morning our team briefly toured a health facility that hadn't been staffed by doctors for several months, since MSF had experienced difficulties in recruiting. Dr. Saied led us on ward rounds, giving advice on the management of the critically ill in-patients to the exhausted medical assistant in charge. We were still cold.

This food-insecure region was extremely poor, with high death rates due to malnourished children. Yet community leaders brought us platters holding two roasted chickens, salty sheep cheese, and cardamom-flavoured coffee to the GTZ project house the next day for our supper. The people here were honoured by our presence and wanted to thank us. Our efforts to pay for the food were refused; our Sudanese counterparts from the government advised we should simply and graciously accept the people's efforts to show thanks. To insist on paying would denigrate their generosity and wound their pride.

Travelling onward, the team settled into an awkward silence, partly in awe at the desert hospitality and partly in anger at the diminishing possibility of pulling a project together that would meet the political needs of both the German and Sudanese governments. The irreconcilable realities had become too visible. Germany wanted to support the war-torn south, having had to end a project in Juba with AMREF when the area became too insecure. Sudan desired more services for the privileged north. It was clear we had been naive to think a compromise might be possible in Darfur, with its mixed population.

Other donor countries had been drawn in by the same illusion of trying to contribute to the rebuilding of poor regions in Sudan. Civil war exacerbates poverty, and in countries such as Sudan the gap can widen between rich and poor. A village of grain silos, proudly marked as development assistance from the government of Italy, served as a testament to misguided or incomplete development. The silos had been built to store grain against further famine. But no top-loading machine had been provided, so there was no mechanism to get grain into the huge containers. For years the shiny silos had stood empty while people tried to think up new useful possibilities, such as turning them on their sides and employing them as rainwater tanks.

At nightfall we came to a huge compound in the desert that housed Italian road builders. Food there was plentiful, accommodations luxurious, and recreation facilities sophisticated. The place required a half-ton of diesel a day to maintain the electricity, water supply, and other utilities. The road would soon be completed, but what would happen to the compound? It would be transferred to the Sudanese government, which would never be able to afford the running costs. Visions of the soon-to-be ghost town enraged me. Of course, the cost of the ongoing war in the south made this fiasco only a minor joke.

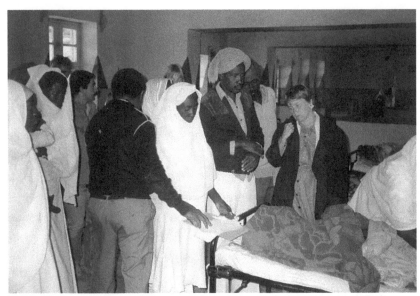

The author visits a small hospital in Darfur, Sudan, accompanied by Sudanese counterparts, a medical assistant, and other staff.

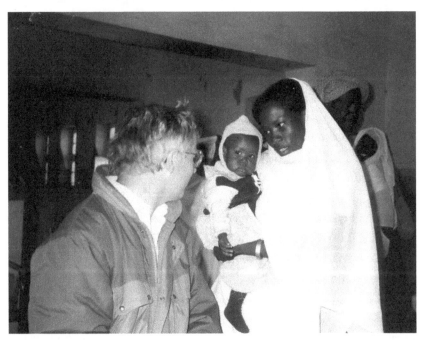

David Porter speaks with a Sudanese nurse and her child in Darfur, Sudan.

Back in Khartoum at our guest house, we discovered that the border was closed. A coup was imminent. The official facilitators from Germany had arrived just before the border shut down. They had come together with their special aluminum project-planning suitcase full of squares of coloured papers and pins to make a visual representation of the problems the project would address. No planes were flying in or out of the country. A curfew was in effect because of rumours of the imminent coup. No one was allowed outside after dusk.

We were confined to the guest house for several days, during which I was ill with alternating vomiting and diarrhea and a severe migraine headache. David gave me a combination of opium, belladonna, and Pepto-Bismol. I took enough to wonder about the possibility of a lifetime supply, and the rest of the mission passed in a happy, drugged haze until I was well enough to join the team as we made a presentation to the Ministry of Health. Throughout our final week we heard screaming military jets coming in at night to protect the government in case of a coup. Accordingly, we clandestinely broke curfew and drove on back streets to a Greek hotel in town that Jens Hasfeldt remembered from a previous trip. This was the only accessible place from which we could phone relatives to say we were safe.

Two days later foreigners and affluent Sudanese were once again allowed to leave. I watched wistfully as Jens and the other Europeans boarded a Lufthansa flight, having booked myself on a much cheaper one on Egypt Air. My plane was delayed for several hours.

As I lined up for the return journey, passengers were separated by gender for boarding. I stood with the kohl-eyed Muslim women. Veiled, with hennaed hands and feet, they waited peacefully, speaking in hushed voices — a contrast to my own Western irritable impatience. I was dreading the many sleepless and uncomfortable hours ahead. I had spent seven weeks away from my family, frustrated with the evil and incompetence I had seen.

A new woman joined our makeshift group — a nun in a white head cloth and long white dress. She didn't seem out of place with the Muslim women, even when she took out a rosary. The nun knew it would be a long wait, time she could use well to pray "Hail Mary, full of grace."

urneys that are as long as these, maybe I needed to learn from her.
nent forward was slow, but there could be peace in the waiting.[6]

UTH SUDAN, 2015

had really wanted to go to South Sudan. It had been more than twenty-five
years since I had been in Sudan, long before the civil war. For the last
decade I had been speaking with one of the designers of the Muskoka
Initiative, a large Canadian-funded mother-and-child health project, which
had organized the South Sudan support. South Sudan was a post-conflict
country with possibly the worst death rates of pregnant women in the
world. I was so excited that Canada had provided substantial aid to mother-
and-child health in this country. For years I had been following the NGOs
working there, such as AMREF. Any chance I got, I would speak to the
Canadian government specialist who had helped set it up. I called him the
lost Baldwin brother, looking as he did like Alec Baldwin. I had also been in
touch with the Canadian head of AMREF Health Canada. In 2013 I had
been the keynote speaker at an AMREF Health Africa fundraising event
in Toronto called Mamatoto (the Swahili word for Mother Baby), which
had a special fund to train African midwives. One country AMREF Health
Africa worked in was South Sudan. Tragically, they had lost one of their
staff in Juba to the ongoing conflict, but this was crucially important work.
Though frightened, I felt it was vitally important to see how a country like
Canada could help conflict and post-conflict countries.

When hera, a Belgian company that does "health and education research
for action" in developing countries and that I have worked for in the past,
won the contract to evaluate the CAD$2.85 billion "Muskoka" Maternal,
Newborn, and Child Health Initiative, I saw an opportunity, as South Sudan
had been one of the Muskoka Initiative target countries. I took myself down
to Ottawa on the twelve-hour overnight bus from my home in northern
Ontario to meet with Canadian government people in the global health
sector about making South Sudan a focus for our evaluation. There was
reluctant agreement, as long as Canada had no responsibility for me. I had
to make my own travel arrangements and could not travel with Canadian

staff in government vehicles. Staff at hera and I interviewed various security companies on Skype, such as ex-British military and police with satellite phones and weapons. Out of our price range — we had not budgeted for security. We chose an American widow who had been married to a Sudanese man, and her daughter, with one vehicle, cellphones, and a Taser.

The long Air Ethiopia economy-class flight from Toronto to Addis, and then on to Juma, the capital of South Sudan, pulled me quickly back to the tired life I had led in previous global health work. And again, such interesting people I met in an exhausted state. My seatmate to Juma was a boy soldier coming back to work in South Sudan as a paramedic. He had been rescued as a young teen, then brought to Canada and educated. This was his first trip back.

I was met at the airport by my American Sudanese guide. She had bought me a cellphone, and she gave me a quick lesson in currency and safety. Shouting in Arabic, she got me through customs lineups and out into the steaming hot Juba day. It was dry and dusty. The road was cracked and uneven. Many people walked on the side of the street, women carrying coloured plastic water buckets and babies. A few chickens pecked in the grass by the road. On our way to my hotel, we were stopped three times by military police hoping for bribes: our windows were too dark; the guide's sandals were not regulation shoes; and did she have permission to travel? Again in Arabic, she chastised the police, mentioned her own friends who were more senior officers, and we were allowed to continue on our way. The streets were run down: goats, pedestrians, motorcycles, and cars jostled for position on the road.

It was the weekend, and as I was to travel upcountry, by air, at the start of the week, *inshallah*, or Allah willing, I wanted to see the hospital in Juba so I could make comparisons with what would be smaller health facilities in the more remote areas. No problem — my American Sudanese guide had often visited the hospital, and she had friends who were senior government officials. She would accompany me safely. I stowed my carry-on bags in the hotel, which reminded me on check-in that I had to pay cash only. I was carrying a lot of cash, debit and credit cards being non -functional in a conflict country.

Off we went to the 580-bed Juba Teaching Hospital. Though it was the weekend, a couple of midwifery tutors were there, preparing lessons and talking with students. Canada had helped to fund midwifery training, so this was a good chance to learn informally how this was going and what some of the difficulties were. I asked one midwifery tutor how she was enjoying her work.

> We are happy there is funding for the students, but it is getting harder to get girls to enrol — many students are males. Women do not have the right qualifications. Families are less likely to pay for education for girls. And then women will not be comfortable having a man as a midwife. Also, we have volunteer midwives from the UN to help us teach. But when the fighting starts, they have to go back to UN safe houses. Some have to leave the country until things get better. But when I started here, the country had only one midwife. Now we have taught over one hundred. If we have peace, this will be a big help for our country. If the fighting continues, those midwives will leave for other countries, like Uganda.

I asked where this midwife had trained. She had worked in Khartoum before the civil war. She had been trained in Arabic and was now teaching in English.

> Many midwives in the northern border states with practical skills in the system do not speak English, though this is now the official language of the country. All midwives in Canadian-supported midwifery institutes are trained in English. This can be difficult as many areas are Arabic speaking and many other health workers have been trained in Arabic. Some Arabic-speaking midwifery students, for example, at the National Training Institute in Wau, have been given a foundation course in English of three months, largely taught by volunteers from the Kenya battalion of peacekeepers.

This was very positive, in comparison with concerns raised elsewhere in this second edition of *A Doctor's Quest* about child prostitution and UN peacekeepers in South Sudan.

We strolled casually outside the wards, looking into the labour ward, postnatal, and pediatrics. I wanted to get a sense of how busy they were, what kind of volume they experienced, and a general sense of how well-equipped and staffed they were. This would help me make comparisons when I would see the wards that Canada had helped to furnish in hospitals outside the capital.

Some of the simple beds had no mattresses but were full of patients, and there were many patients on the floor. Relatives sat outside, the women in colourful dresses, the men with T-shirts and pants, either barefoot or wearing rubber flip-flops, some trying to prepare food for their ill family members. Two little girls in slightly torn dresses laughed, chasing a ball with a stick outside the door to the ward.

My guide brought me back to my hotel and then suggested we dine overlooking the Nile. I was not expecting such luxury, lovely food, and a fine setting with a beautiful view. The ongoing violence seemed very remote. We arranged for her to pick me up in the morning, to quickly meet my counterparts in the Canadian Embassy, then to travel upcountry.

Previously, the only flights had been UNMISS (UN Mission) flights, for UN staff and selected bilateral government employees. I was not allowed to be considered an official Canadian representative, so could not fly on those flights. I was an external independent consultant. Fortunately, a private-sector carrier from South Africa had just started to run limited flights, and I was able to get a seat on one of those. The health adviser from the Canadian Embassy accompanied me, and my American Sudanese driver had arranged our transport in the field through some other freelance companies that could drive us to health facilities and non-governmental organizations providing health services. There had been some debate where we could go, as the shifting borders of insecurity kept changing which places were safe for travel.

South Sudan is the newest country in the world after decades of civil war that killed 2.5 million people, displaced 4 million people, and destroyed much of the country's physical infrastructure. The population is estimated at 10.9 million, which is more than 90 percent rural, and nearly 90 percent of women are illiterate. Over half the population has negligible access to health care. It is one of the poorest countries in the world (half the population lives on less than one dollar a day), and maternal mortality ratios are among the highest globally. The 2006 South Sudan Household Health Survey stated that 2,054 women died per 100,000 live births, at that time the highest in the world. Estimates vary widely. The World Bank has also cited 789 per 100,000 livebirths for maternal mortality ratio. This is the latest year for which we have maternal mortality data. Canada had funded a maternal mortality survey, but it had not yet been done at the time of our visit because of the insecurity in the country, which restricted travel.[7] Wasting, or acute malnutrition in children under five, was over 10 percent in South Sudan, one of only fourteen countries to have this level.

The 2018 Fragile States Index ranked South Sudan as the most fragile state in the world. The decades-long civil conflict left weak governance. After only three years of peace, an internal struggle in the Sudan Liberation People's Movement led to the December 2013 conflict that resulted in fifty thousand dead, 1.9 million displaced within South Sudan, and one hundred thousand sheltering in UN bases. Almost half a million people fled to neighbouring countries. Further famines were to follow. And since 2015, when I was there, ongoing conflict and civil war worsened the situation. In South Sudan as of 2017, 1.5 million refugees have left, and there is ongoing genocide, rape, and famine.[8]

What had Canada and other countries offering aid tried to do? Canada committed $72.8 million towards mother, newborn, and child health in South Sudan over five years, a huge increase in support from a very low base before the Muskoka Initiative.

Since contraception is the most cost-effective way to save the lives of pregnant women and children under five, this was a large part of our support. However, Canada, from 2006 to 2015 had a Conservative prime minister, and family planning would not appeal to his political base. Still, although the Muskoka health program designers were able to provide contraceptive commodity support through the UN, only 6 percent of women had access to birth control. Rape was, and continues to be, common. More than one in ten children die before they are five. Canada helped to finance research through NGOs that showed simply trained community health workers with a basic medicine kit could treat the major causes of death: malaria, pneumonia, and diarrhea. Integrated community case management is now endorsed by UNICEF and the World Health Organization as a cost-effective strategy in low-income settings, including conflict and post-conflict countries. The Countdown to 2030 strategy cites interventions such as these that can be delivered at the community level to be more equitable than those requiring access to fixed and equipped facilities.

I spoke with one of the NGO workers that Canada supported in South Sudan, with additional financing from the Global Fund:

> Our coalition of NGOs provided life-saving treatment for well over three million children, with a total of 3,221,916 treatments given by the community drug distributors across the integrated community case management package of malaria, pneumonia, and diarrhea. But then Canada decided to withdraw support. We risked losing the Global Fund grant and ending this life-saving intervention. Several of us NGOs sent an urgent position paper to the Canadian government.

Still, when for unclear political reasons Canada decided to withdraw this support, advocacy with other donors ensured that Britain's Department for International Development was able to pick this up to sustain such an important initiative. Canada did support, with other countries, immunization — only 10 percent of children under two had been immunized.

The results in South Sudan led to reductions in the deaths of children under five and infants under one. And importantly, Canada trained more than one hundred midwives and helped improve the skills for emergency obstetric care by training non-specialists to do Caesarean sections (C-sections). But still only 15 percent of women had access to a skilled birth attendant, and most of these were more affluent women.

A real constraint is the lack of trained health workers. There are only 1.5 physicians and 2 nurses/midwives for every 100,000 citizens, mostly in urban areas, according to the South Sudan Health Sector Development Plan

2012–16. Only 10 percent of health positions are filled with appropriately trained workers according to the Inventory Survey of Human Resources for Health in Southern Sudan 2006. Canada not only helped train health workers but also helped distribute them. Government wages are lower than salaries in the NGO sector. Recruitment in the public sector has therefore been difficult. Canada was a key player in a move to harmonize salaries, including through the introduction of an extra allowance for staff in hard-to-reach areas, an allowance paid since January 2015 as an advance, as salaries are often not paid on time.

When we arrived by air to an upcountry region supported by Canadian assistance, we had plans to meet with small clinics as well as a district hospital. We met first with the senior doctor at the hospital:

> We are grateful that Canada has helped equip our theatre for us to be able to do Caesarean sections. Canada, through the UN, trained the doctors to provide emergency obstetric care. This was called "task-shifting" so we don't have to wait for specialist obstetricians but someone who is more quickly trained to provide this service. But still we have big problems. Many women die of post-partum hemorrhage.

Canada helped to determine specific problems that could be addressed. An emergency obstetric and neonatal care assessment funded by Canada was conducted by the Ministry of Health, with United Nations Population Fund (UNFPA) assistance in October 2013. One issue addressed was the problem of post-partum hemorrhage. Even countries that have really improved the health of pregnant women and children under five, such as Bhutan, have found this to be a major problem because of lack of access to important medicines and midwifery skills to control bleeding after childbirth. In South Sudan a strategy was developed to combine activities to support active management of the third stage of labour and provision of oxytocin (given by needle) for facility births, with misoprostol (which can be given rectally) for home births (to control and prevent hemorrhage) — a strategy developed and implemented by UNFPA, bilateral donors, WHO, NGOs, and the Government of South Sudan.

One problem in South Sudan is a large inequity in access to health care. In 2012, almost 60 percent of health care costs were paid by people out of pocket, 30 percent came from countries like Canada as development assistance, and less than 10 percent came from domestic sources or the government of South Sudan. In 2016 it was estimated that South Sudan spent 25 percent or more of its own government money on war — displacing health and education.[9] The ongoing conflict has had several effects. Many upgraded facilities that Canada had financed were wasted as the civil war kept shifting boundaries, meaning hospitals were now in conflict zones and could not be utilized. And though Canada had paid to improve the facilities, military spending by the South Sudan government meant that hospital costs and salaries were not paid.

As our visits to the shiny new facilities revealed, too few were being used. Fuel to keep operating rooms air-conditioned had not been paid for. Hostels for pregnant women awaiting delivery were empty because no one had money for food. Staff had not had salaries paid. Was this corruption at the national or state level?

The problem of military spending is not unique to South Sudan. The Stockholm International Peace Institute estimated in April 2017 that total global military expenditure rose in 2016 to $1,686 billion.[10] In South Sudan over 10 percent of their gross domestic product was spent on the military. But this was a decrease: South Sudan expenditures fell 54 percent and Saudi Arabia by 30 percent as their national oil revenues fell, one of the reasons for the ongoing conflict being the fight over access to oil.

The recent *Lancet* review, "Countdown to 2030: Tracking Progress Towards Universal Coverage for Reproductive, Maternal, Newborn, and Child Health" (by the Countdown to 2030 Collaboration) has developed a system to monitor progress in the eighty-one countries that account for 95 percent of maternal deaths and 90 percent of child deaths worldwide. Just as the Millennium Development Goals tracked progress to 2015, this new challenge tracks achievements toward the Sustainable Development Goals. A strengthened focus is how to support women and children in conflict settings such as South Sudan. South Sudan is one of ten Countdown countries that has experienced severe conflicts from 2011 to 2016 — defined as five thousand battle-related deaths and more than one hundred thousand refugees, asylum seekers, and internally displaced people in 2016. Globally, most internally displaced people are women and children. Women and girls are also the victims of sexual violence. Canada's support to South Sudan, though difficult, was an important contribution to developing strategies for assisting conflict countries in reproductive, maternal, newborn, and child health.

And even in 2015, in hera's Formative Evaluation of Canada's Contribution to the Maternal, Newborn and Child Health (MNCH) Initiative, the inequities in access to reproductive, maternal, newborn, and child health services were glaring. Wealthy women in South Sudan in 2010 — the top income quintile (68 percent) — were three times more likely than poor women or the bottom economic quintile (22 percent) to have one prenatal visit. Aggregated (all income quintiles) data showed that only 17 percent of all women had four prenatal visits, WHO's recommended minimum. Forty percent of wealthy women and eight percent of poor women have a skilled birth attendant such as a midwife at their deliveries. The majority have an untrained birth attendant such as a family member, or they deliver alone.

These inequities will be further exacerbated as conflict continues, though monitoring of health service utilization will become more difficult. Canada's support in training over one hundred midwives was very important. Very few women at any income level had access to emergency obstetric care (1.8 percent of wealthy women and 0.2 percent of the poor) and less than 10 percent at any income level had access to contraception. Canada's support in equipping operating rooms to provide Caesarean sections and train non-specialists to do emergency obstetric care was highly relevant. Very few women of any income level had access to contraception, around 10 percent. Child health data shows that poor women (50 percent) were more likely to initiate breastfeeding than wealthy women (40 percent), but other indicators such as immunization, vitamin A drops to improve immunity, oral rehydration, and insecticide-treated bed nets show wealthy families were two to four times more likely to get these services (South Sudan Household Health Survey 2010). Again, this shows the importance of integrated community case management of childhood illness, where quickly trained informal health workers with basic medicines can treat the common causes of childhood illness and death in low resource settings such as South Sudan.

After our visits to the field, hospitals, health facilities, non-governmental organizations, and community groups, we prepared to fly back to the capital. But now the air traffic controllers were on strike, because their salaries had not been paid. My colleague called United Nations Mission in South Sudan. Could we get on a UNMISS flight? Could I have permission to fly on it? The answer was yes on both counts, and I still treasure my scanned emailed note allowing me on that flight, even though I did not take it. We covered both bases, lining up at the airport in case the strike ended and commercial flights could go.

———

I was again reminded of my first trip to Sudan, in 1989, when the lines to board were separated by gender. A shout went out — yes, the plane was going to be allowed to fly to Juba. The flight was overbooked — first come, first served. The men were allowed to board. Families were separated, women and children in the other line. I was furious. We had been waiting longer than many of these men. Not speaking Arabic, I was shrill and powerless. The men helping to board shrugged. We could not get on the plane until a woman was found who could search us. Somehow, we made it onto the plane, took off, and arrived to even more than the usual chaos in Juba. My Sudanese American guide met me and sadly advised me that one of her neighbours had been killed the night before. Although he had not been out past curfew, he was attacked as he arrived at home early in the evening.

In Khartoum in 1989, our team had travelled to Omdurman, to the Hamed al-Nil tomb to watch the whirling dervish dancing. This is a Sufi Muslim ascetic sect, who dress in green and white and dance and spin and clap while shouting, "*La illaha illallah*" (There is no God but Allah). The word *dervish* is derived from an old Persian word and translates as someone who goes door to door, singing, and seeking alms for the poor. The development dance is a whirling dervish of its own, spinning and trying to get money for the poor, but the dance careens out of control too often, and the hand of God or Allah is very hard to see.

2

I Do Not Have the Freedom
That You Have as a Woman:

Bangladesh, Nepal, Ghana,
and a Global Reflection

Bangladesh, 1990

We arrived at the round thatch-roofed house constructed of mud, sticks, and manure. I, the only woman, entered alone. Jens, the other men on the team, and the male translator sat outside on the step with their backs to the women inside. The Bangladeshi translator had to listen carefully to hear what I was saying and, without turning around, rephrase my words into Bangla and the women's replies into English. I tried to pick up the non-verbal cues of these well-covered women. I asked about childbirth: Did they know anyone who had died? "Yes, it is common." And children, what did they do if they got sick? "For women's illnesses, and for our children, we go to traditional healers. They understand better. We do not have the money to go to the hospital. When we give birth, we go to the traditional birth attendant [TBA]. She will deliver our baby for a small gift, some soap, or rice, or a simple sari. And if we have nothing to give her, she will still help us. But she does not know what to do when things go wrong. She is not accepted at the hospital."

I asked the men of the family who had stayed in the room to observe us if they knew that women needed extra food and special care in pregnancy. "No, we make sure our women do what is expected of them. Pregnancy is no excuse for laziness and special attention. We still have to correct them if they disobey."

By correcting, the men meant beating. I knew that up to 12 percent of the pregnant women who died in Bangladesh died because of violence.[1] I wanted to cry. Progress ending violence against women and the neglect of their needs would indeed be a long and slow journey.

I asked the women if they were afraid of dying in labour. "Yes," they said, looking at me sadly through their veils, "it is common." One husband said it was better to let the wife die and then get a new wife with a new dowry. And children dying, I asked, was that common, too? "Yes," replied the women shyly. One in seven children would die by the age of five in this area. The women's dark eyes were sad but accepting. They asked if I had children. I showed them pictures of my son and daughter. They were happy to see my family. Then they smiled, introduced me to their children, and let me hold them.

With a baby on my hip, I recalled how it felt carrying Anna and Alec when they were small. Later, as we sat cross-legged on the floor together, I was offered bitter betel nut and lime on a palm leaf. I couldn't help but think how unlikely it would be for me to welcome uninvited strangers into my Canadian home, as these women had graciously allowed for us. Would we be so forthcoming discussing childbirth customs, even with a woman, when there were men sitting on the doorstep? We spoke through a translator so that communication was limited to its simplest level through facial expressions and gestures. It was a comfort to relate with a trusting innocence that permitted us as human beings to connect through the heart. In the process of our own development, I fear we have lost that capacity.

When I first arrived in Bangladesh, it took me a moment to understand why everything seemed so strange — over 90 percent of the people around me were men. In 1990 you seldom saw a woman on the street or in a rickshaw unless she was with her husband, father, brother, or elder son. Or if she was a single parent, she might be seen doing hard labour, breaking old bricks into gravel to make roads.

I was on a five-week assignment to help strengthen NGOs working with mother-and-child health. After we worked together in Sudan, Jens had asked me to join his small co-operative of international health consultants based in Copenhagen and to work with him on an assignment in Bangladesh — a trip that required three uncomfortable days of travel overwhelmed by the reek of urine in the splattered economy-class toilets and the total exhaustion of no sleep from Toronto to London to Delhi to Dhaka.

The security situation was very unstable, rife with *hartals* (strikes) and street violence. Police in riot gear clubbed protesters with sticks. I was also adjusting to the intensity of the population pressure in Asia, which felt quite different from what I had encountered in Africa. I had become used to the easy grace of Africans; things moved more slowly there. The insistent bustle of Dhaka unnerved me.

Diesel fumes assaulted my nose and eyes as I searched for the prearranged car to bring me to the guest house. Most of the people crowding around me were men, who constantly spat, save for a few mothers with sick-looking babies in their arms. These women showed their hunger by placing empty hands to their mouths with imploring eyes while they begged for coins.

It was a welcome relief to travel away from Bangladesh's capital to a southeastern region. En route our small group — three Bangladeshis who included two health workers and a translator, and Jens and I — managed a brief stop by the Bay of Bengal, where we picked our way across sand dunes covered with morning glories. The strong surf from the bay pounded the shore, while tall palm trees towered over small homes nestled beneath. The fine salty spray tingled slightly on our faces and teased our noses.

Our team had come to this small village as part of a primary health-care project whose goal was to improve the health of mothers and children in the area. The project included simple interventions that could save the most lives: immunizing children and monitoring growth to ensure good nutrition, treating common illnesses such as diarrhea and pneumonia, providing prenatal care and safe delivery care, ensuring an adequate supply of essential drugs, and improving water and sanitation. In order to design the project we had to first assess the current situation by visiting homes and health facilities, as well as reviewing the statistics to see what level of care was available and where there were gaps.

We learned from many women that they were slowly developing the confidence to move outside their secluded family roles. That had been unheard of before health workers started going door to door to see female patients who were often not allowed out of their homes to seek health care. But through NGO as well as government projects, these women were now learning to read, to speak out, and to go to the health centre when they or their children were sick. We met with community members who told us, "Now we can travel on our own to the health centre. We move in groups of three. We still wear our burkas, but the men accept that we can move without our husbands to accompany us." These dignified women made me look within myself. I had chosen poverty with my family when my husband was working with Indigenous Peoples' land claims in Canada, but I knew it was something we could easily change. I had faced complications in labour and delivery, especially with my daughter, Anna. But even though my journey then involved boat travel and a broken-down car on isolated roads for several hours, I was able to reach a hospital and emergency obstetric care that saved my life from a post-partum hemorrhage and my daughter's from a hypoglycemic coma. And we had paid nothing for that service. These women faced the risks of giving birth, with a family member or friend, and no hope of medical support for any problems they might face. Still, we were united as women who had given birth. We connected heart to heart, eye to eye. One traditional birth attendant, Shireen, spoke through a translator. "These women struggle to save twenty taka a month [then about seventy-five cents] to pay for a safer childbirth. Today they have dressed in their finest clothes to greet us. They are honoured that we are visiting them in their own community."

Shefali was one of the women. She wore a black hooded burka. She explained how she had lost two sisters in childbirth, two of her own children had died from pneumonia, and her mother-in-law still blamed her for the deaths of the children. I could barely see her eyes, but her voice was shaking to hold back the tears she was too proud to show.

Shireen wasn't in such conservative dress. As a health worker, she wore a *shalwar kameez*, which was still acceptable for a woman and allowed her more mobility to see her community in door-to-door visits. She explained, "Many mothers and babies used to die during childbirth. But now, because we are better trained as a result of this combined government and NGO health project, deaths are fewer. Still, in a hard labour, if the mother has no money for transport to a health centre [about two hundred taka — ten times what she is able to save in a month] or for medical expenses, she will often die." Each of these aides delivered anywhere from four to more than fifty babies over a six-month period. They often lacked money to buy soap to wash their hands before a delivery, or for the blades to cut the cord.

Shireen went on to emphasize: "We must do this work. It is hard to leave our families to help the women, but we must. We usually work for no money, maybe for a little soap or some clothing. Once, I was faced with a woman who was slowly bleeding to death, and I had to remove the afterbirth — which was stuck inside her — with my bare hands. Last year in this very village, to save the life of a mother I had to cut an unborn baby into pieces when it got stuck in the birth canal. I had to tell her family that both their daughter and grandson had died despite my sleepless night trying to deliver them by candlelight alone. I hope I never have to do that again in my life. That memory weighs too heavily on my heart."

Shireen and other TBAs I met had handled more difficult deliveries than I had, with my longer and more professional training. They had remained strong and committed to their work even if mothers or children died because greater technical help was out of reach.

Ironically, traditional birth attendants like Shireen didn't meet the WHO standards of "skilled birth attendant." She wasn't able to get training, while midwives got their skills upgraded. However, the ones with university education didn't stay in these poor villages, or even in Bangladesh. They left for good jobs in the Middle East.

Equality with men will always be elusive. What man faces death bringing life into the world?

Jens and I passed along the coast and then travelled inland through rice paddies. Lining the roads were a few water buffalo and scrawny cattle with white egrets riding on their backs. We had been happy to plan for improved health care for these coastal villages, with better training for the traditional birth attendants and a referral system so that women with complications could be accompanied by a birth attendant and brought to a health centre. It was good to see the strengths in these villages, the dedication of women helping one another for little or no material reward.

In my heart I knew how hard it was for these women to leave their homes. In many ways their walk of a few miles mirrored my own much longer journey. I, too, had to tear myself away from my family to travel to Uganda, Sudan, and Bangladesh. This was the beginning of my obsession with the lives of poor women in distant lands, women I could help as a doctor even if I had to go thousands of miles to find them. At home in Canada I could hear them calling, hear their voices in the wind telling me I was needed and I must follow.

NEPAL, 1991

In Bangladesh, women in a largely Muslim society were moving slowly out of their limited roles in their family compound, with little access to reproductive health services except contraception. Half of the women in Bangladesh used family planning, the cheapest way to save women's lives during pregnancy.[2] But in Nepal, a largely Hindu and Buddhist society, access to contraceptives was more limited. Here, too, women delivered at home and had few midwives or hospitals to go to for emergencies. And in Nepal, as in Bangladesh, women were very much seen as an underclass.

In March 2008 a U.K. Maternal Health Parliamentarian Forum[3] cited Nepal as one of the successful models in its halving of maternal deaths when access to skilled attendants, emergency obstetric care, family planning, and safe abortion were improved.[4] Less than twenty years earlier, abortion was a major cause of maternal deaths.[5] In 1991, I watched helplessly as Sunita died. Her parents told us she hadn't wanted another child, but her husband insisted on the pregnancy, hoping for a son instead of a fourth unwanted daughter.

Women didn't get to choose when they had sex. Rape was common. They often couldn't get contraception. But in every village someone knew how to abort a pregnancy with herbs or twigs. So a woman with no income and low status, with an unwanted pregnancy, had to resort to a clandestine abortion. Sunita had arrived at the hospital in septic shock, dying. She had travelled hours by ox cart but arrived too late, and there weren't enough antibiotics to save her.

On the heels of the Bangladesh project, with a bare three days home between missions, I came to Nepal in 1991 to join a Canadian International Development Agency (CIDA) health project team comprised of both Nepalis and Canadians. We were being sent to a remote district — where a woman had a one-in-twelve chance of dying in labour in her lifetime — to evaluate the improvements of community development.

A stomach-churning ride through the mountains northwest of the capital city and a six-hour walk were required to reach one of the health project villages in the valley near Surkhet. The twisting roads didn't help the onset of one of my migraines, made worse by jet lag, but the extraordinary scenery that unfolded before me was an enormous distraction. Found in the same pocket of the universe as Bangladesh, Nepal seemed a world away.

Huge banks of marigolds framed the sky, while in the distance, beyond the flowers, high mountains shimmered in the clear, thin air. Closer to us, simple homes clustered in tiny villages. Compared with the women with scarlet imprints on their foreheads and brightly patterned cotton blouses and long, flowing skirts, the men were plainer, dressed in beige and grey-brown garments and close-fitting hats. We stood aside on the mountain path for a young girl, already married at thirteen, who was herding goats.

The people and animals lived so closely together that women gave birth in a barn with the water buffalo. Most women had delivered at least one baby, helping their sisters or their daughters. Many were highly skilled in deliveries. The scents of smoke from wood fires and brewing tea mixed together in the cold mountain air.

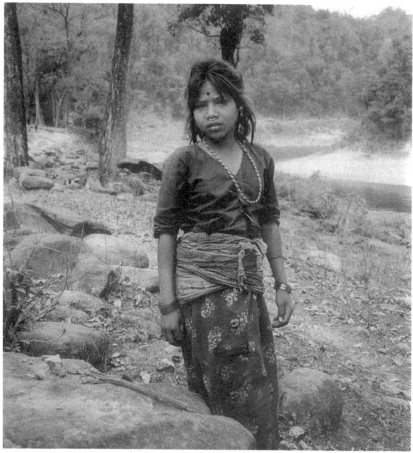

A young married girl herds goats in rural Nepal.

To keep these fires burning, women and girls carried huge loads of branches on their back, surely contributing to the sight of so many trees stripped of every branch and twig, silent evidence of the deforestation in Nepal that contributes to soil erosion and floods in Bangladesh.

It was night when we arrived in the health project village. The outer walls of the wooden homes were plastered with white mud. Women sat cross-legged before their doorways, their long vivid skirts wrapped around them, while chickens and goats foraged in the sand. Children stood sadly next to a mud wall.

The porters who carried our bags had arrived hours ahead of us and had tea and *dahl baht* (the ubiquitous lentils and rice) waiting for us. Pleading ill health, I retreated early to a sleeping bag in a loft room. But really it was because I needed to be alone. Too many strange images had confounded me.

Traversing the mountain earlier that day, we had peered into a valley below on the other side that could have been Shangri-La with its explosion of colours and blankets of marigolds. Suddenly, we heard drumming and chanting and cleared a path for a procession coming toward us. What was this? The only ones in the march were men, winding into sight one by one around the bend, following the leader who played a mournful drum.

There was a hush among us. Then we saw the bier carrying the draped, red-cloth-covered body of a pregnant woman. We were told she had died in labour. This was her funeral procession curving downhill from us and around to the next bend. The drumming faded away as the last person rounded the corner and vanished out of sight. The intense sunlight left us dazzled and dismayed. We stood still, silent, humbled. This was the most poignant reminder of why we were here.

Now, in the darkness, I heard the rustle of rats moving through the walls. As I recalled the procession marking the loss of two lives, I was close to crying. With unshed tears stinging my eyes, I finally fell asleep.

In the morning our mixed Nepali and Canadian public health team met with the community and sat under spreading branches in a clearing, attending a village meeting while goats strolled among us. A light wind rattled through huge dry leaves above our heads. Men and women lined separate sides of the circle and took turns discussing their problems and achievements. The women were proud of their improved reading skill, the savings and credit groups they had formed, and their ability to weave and sell the clothing they made to earn extra income for their families. The men were working to help irrigate the land and seemed to accept the women, who formerly had never spoken at such a public meeting. It was impressive to witness such an effective example of community development, which, though funded by Canada, had been catalyzed by Nepali leaders at the village level.

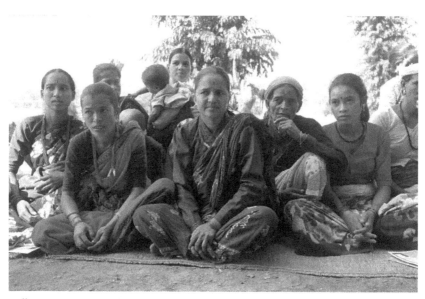

Village women in Surkhet, Nepal.

The project had carefully trained women to make smokeless *chulos*, or cookstoves, which burned less wood and caused less smoke to fill the small homes. This helped to reduce chest infections. Other villagers from far away had been so interested in these activities that they had walked several days to attend the meeting, and later stayed to find out how they could implement these improvements in their own communities.

In addition to this and other village gatherings, we saw patients in the project house and health centre, where small children showed us marigolds that they clutched tightly in their curled hands. Everywhere we were greeted with garlands of marigolds placed over our heads and were given individual blossoms to hold.

In one community we saw improvements in the small hospital, now better able to manage complicated cases that would previously have required expensive referral or led to death. Here we met Tahera, who was twelve years old and in an arranged marriage. Tahera's hips were too small for early child-bearing. We saw her moments after she arrived in hospital, moments before she died with an obstructed labour. There was no one with the skill or equipment to do a Caesarean section, and she had come too late. Although trained to do Caesarean sections, doctors feared reprisals if they made mistakes. Through lack of practice, they quickly lost these skills.

We met women who had walked the long distances between their rural villages and health-care facilities, since there were poor or non-existent methods of transport for patients. In one village we met Shushir, a husband who didn't allow his wife, Ali, to leave home for a hospital delivery, even though she was hemorrhaging in labour. His reason: because she had to feed the water buffalo. "Her duty is to stay here. If she dies, it is fated and I will get a new wife and a new dowry." The wife didn't question him. Luckily, in this case, the local health worker had medicine to control the bleeding, so Ali didn't die. In Africa, as well, I had seen the low value put on women's lives, but in Africa there is a bride price, so a man has to buy a wife (in cattle, for example). In many parts of Asia, the dowry system means that fathers have to pay to get rid of their daughters through marriage.

One woman explained that they eat less during pregnancy than normal, hoping for a smaller baby and an easier delivery. Women traditionally eat least and last in any case, giving the best food to their husbands and sons. She added that she ate soil during pregnancy. "We are hungry. Our husbands say we already have something in our bellies, so they take what food there is, and we must eat soil to fill our hunger." While in some cultures the women eat dirt during pregnancy to obtain scarce nutrients such as iron, these undernourished women were simply trying to obtain a sensation of fullness. By the time they gave birth, they were so anemic at delivery that even a slight blood loss could lead to death.

Through it all I was overwhelmed by the richness and stunned by the intensity of these encounters with poor women. I was doing challenging work, was saddened to have left my husband and children twice in such a short period, ached to see my eleven-year-old daughter and eight-year-old son, and was still recovering from the violence I had seen in Dhaka. This combination meant that I often had to isolate myself while enduring another migraine in yet another village home while a solicitous Nepali Samaritan brought me bananas and tea, nourishing my body and my spirit. These women were so strong. They carried so many burdens — hauling heavy loads on their backs, looking after their children, working from long before dawn until late at night, eating very little food. And they were now helping to carry me.

During our return journey to Kathmandu, we had trouble crossing a river to a town from which we were to begin an eight-hour walking trip. We saw a raft of foreigners, one who turned out to be a Canadian we'd met on the plane — an engineer in an Australian wide-brimmed hat. We begged a lift across the river and chatted about a wildlife count he was doing before the river was flooded to make hydroelectric power. After breakfasting on huge cucumber slices and yoghurt, we set off again for two more days of walking. In the villages we passed on foot, always unannounced, we were stopped and welcomed — once with hot yak milk, once with lassi.

As if through newly opened eyes, I now saw child wives and women doubled over with firewood as a normal part of the landscape. I had lost my outrage. I had slowed to the pace of change that would be needed. I was flowing through the currents of women's lives that were extraordinarily different from my own. The children sold into marriage to pay off a family debt, the women who were not given enough to eat, who had a one-in-twelve chance of dying when they were pregnant. I wasn't sure if I was bending to make the disturbing scenes I was witnessing easier for my soul, or if this ability to be fluid was to make my work more effective. This continues to be a struggle. It is a challenging balance to be angry and aware enough to fight for change, and still be patient in order to accept that change will come so slowly.

In our visit to the village where we were to sleep on our last night, we women were allowed the first chance to bathe. So down the stony path we went in the dark, feeling our way carefully by flashlight to the river, cool and refreshing on our tired, dusty bodies. The Nepalis in our group bathed with their clothes on, around the bend from us, laughing shyly. The rushing water bubbled over the rocks, and we three Canadians in the group found hollows to lie in that just fit our naked backs. Bare trees glowed eerily grey-green on the other side of the riverbank, dim in the quickly falling night. I lay down in the current and watched playful fireflies as golden as the marigolds.

At night again, under the stars in my sleeping bag on the veranda, all the contradictions began to sort themselves out. I gazed up at the night sky, seeing new constellations, bright night stars connecting in new patterns like the knowledge and confidence of the village women. I could still feel the delicious wetness on my skin from the river and hear the rushing as the water wound across the stones. The process of change was so slow. It took many months to teach health workers to save women's lives, and it was even more difficult to change long-held attitudes in communities so they would value these women who faced death so bravely. But just as the stars pierced the vast blackness of the night sky, the glimmer of progress kept me motivated, kept me working toward the light. As I fell asleep, the sweet bitter scent of bright marigolds drifted through my dreams.

GHANA, 1992

We passed a woman walking slowly. She was carrying what appeared to be a fifty-pound load on her head, a baby on her back, and a child at her side. Her husband rode his bicycle beside her, carrying nothing. We stopped, and Jens leaned out. "Can we help? Do you want a lift?"

He spoke to the woman in English. She cast her eyes down. Joe, our Ghanaian driver, got out of the driver's side and asked in Dagaare, "Can we help you?"

Furious, her husband pushed his wife and son ahead of him and tried to insert himself in the car, throwing his bike onto the roof rack. "Just drop me near the Uplands Hotel. She can walk. It isn't far."

He spoke in perfect English. We looked at one another. Jens said, "No, sir. I offered the lift to your wife. She has the heavier load."

The man replied, "Either I take the lift, or she'll be beaten for causing me this embarrassment."

We drove on with him in our car, none of us speaking, as his wife trudged slowly behind us with their children.

In rural Ghana back then, half as many girls as boys had an education, a disparity that continues.[6] Most girls became pregnant when they were teenagers. Adolescents had a higher risk of dying in labour, so these young girls with no income, totally dependent on their husband's family, were unable to obtain enough money to be cared for if they had an emergency delivery. In a Christian and Muslim society, in Sub-Saharan Africa, this region of Upper West had the poorest quality prenatal care and the least access to skilled birth attendants in Ghana. Here, there was very little available family planning. These regional differences have persisted.[7]

I had come to Ghana in 1992 to work with Jens Hasfeldt again, this time on a project funded by the Danish government. It combined the training of community nurse midwives with support to Ghana's poorest region, Upper West, in the north on the Burkina Faso border. We were a team of four: Jens, the overall project manager; Lise Kaalund, a Danish public health nurse; myself, a public health doctor; and our driver, Joe, who loved to play gospel music.

It was a long journey from Accra to Wa, the capital of Upper West. We passed isolated villages of a few huts moulded out of red earth and cow dung, chickens scampering in the dirt outside searching for grain. We drove for as long as an hour at a time without seeing any living thing.

In Kumasi we stopped at a market to load up on supplies. The women traders of Ghana were bustling and enterprising, shouting out competitive prices as they stood beside piles of brilliant vegetables and fruit. Carefully balanced pyramids of tomatoes perched beside onions, rush bags of eggs leaned against displays of ground nuts, and bananas smelled sweet and inviting. We bought bags of them as well as cookies for the road and spaghetti for a quick dinner later.

After Kumasi the tarmac disappeared, as did the towns and the occasional car. We made another rest stop in a Lobi village not far from Wa. The Lobi and the Wala tribes are linked historically. The Lobi have a tradition of inserting plates in women's lower lips. Joe, acting as our translator, enabled us to greet the villagers. Three women came to meet us. Two stood with their hoes in the millet garden, and one carried a wide metal bowl full of grain on her head. All of them had dusty bare feet and wore dirty Western clothing, in contrast to their traditional look with the bottom gums missing two teeth, the better to show off their plated lips. They stood in front of an ochre-coloured clay home. Two smiling kids played at their feet, necks garlanded with beads, brown bodies naked, bellies distended, most likely with worms.

Joe was curious. "What is that?" he asked in the local dialect, pointing to a scrap of white material fluttering from the roof of the dwelling next door.

The women glanced shyly away and laughed. "That man has captured a woman. Those are her underclothes. He is warning her husband that he has her now and is daring him to try to take her back." Goats wandered by us, bored. The sun warmed our faces as we listened to Joe and the women, waiting for Joe to translate the conversation back to us. Crickets sang in the grass, and the leaves flapped and fluttered in the breeze. I could hear two distinct songs: a steady musical hum and a low trilling.

"She is a lucky one," the tallest of the three women said. "He is a great man. He has many cows. She will be a happy junior bride. His wives obey him. He seldom has to beat them."

Jens laughed, then stopped when Lise and I shot him stern looks. "Okay, enough. Let's move on." Jens led us back to our Rover, and we waved goodbye.

Joe shifted back from translator to driver and turned the gospel music back on, and we set off amid a cloud of dust.

A battered yellow taxi loaded with bundles, bags, and boxes tied to its roof sat stalled in the middle of the road. The hood was open. A short, sturdy man about five feet, six inches tall stood in loose trousers and a blue T-shirt, gazing hopefully at the engine. There was a woman with a young boy at her side beside the man, who I assumed was her husband.

Jens and Joe got out of our car and strode purposefully over to the taxi. Lise and I stayed inside, chatting quietly, glancing occasionally at the men standing around the taxi who poked at the wiring authoritatively. The men took turns trying to start the engine. Only an occasional grumbling cough was heard followed by sheepish silence and the screaming of bush shrikes.

After forty minutes, Lise abruptly opened the door and stomped over to the taxi. "Okay, guys, out." She played with the fuses on the front dash and moved a few around tentatively. The engine started, then rumbled steadily. "Okay!" she said, turning to the blue-shirted man and his family. "You won't have lights, so get in and drive quickly so you get to Wa before it gets too dark. But the engine will be fine. Just get more fuses tomorrow so you can have both lights and engine." The man turned to Jens and thanked him. He ignored Lise entirely. What was it about women in Ghana that made them invisible to men? How could women just be bought and sold between men? How could men treat women as though they were slaves? Why was a man being thanked for the work done by a woman?

It was 9:00 p.m. when we finally arrived at the guest house in Wa. The generator was throbbing in the rear courtyard. We each had a simple room with a small wooden bed. I quickly prepared a late supper of spaghetti and tomato sauce from the provisions we had bought on the way. Tomorrow we could go down the road to the Ghanaian outdoor restaurant with wooden chairs and tables under the trees, which served goat or guinea fowl. Jens had taught the woman who ran the restaurant how to make avocado vinaigrette. Already my mouth was watering, thinking of that avocado under the trees at dusk.

The next morning, after a quick breakfast, we stopped at the Regional Health Management Team headquarters. We picked up two nurses, Georgina and Basilia, who would travel with us to visit more remote districts. Jens and Lise stayed at the headquarters to discuss the overall project management with the regional director.

It was many exhausting, bouncing hours later that Basilia, Georgina, and I arrived in Tumu district. We entered a village of perhaps forty homes, an hour by road from the district hospital. In one *rondavel* we heard shouted screams. We stopped. Someone sounded in terrible pain — could we help? We poked our heads through the simple opening. Basilia spoke in Sisaala, "We are health workers. What can we do to help?" A young pregnant woman was writhing in labour, holding on to a rope above her head. She was squatting and had angry red welts on her arms.

"We do not need your help," her family replied in their own language to Basilia, who translated for me. A man and two women were beating her with branches. Her husband? Sister and mother-in-law? "She has misbehaved. She has been with another man who has made her pregnant. She must confess or the baby will not come."

Basilia and Georgina quickly explained, "No, she is too small. This has nothing to do with who the father of the baby is. She is innocent of adultery. How old is she? Thirteen? Fourteen? The baby is stuck inside her. She needs help. Maybe an operation. We can bring her to the hospital. How long has she been in labour? Fifteen hours? That's too long. Let us examine her."

I moved outside. I wasn't needed here. I didn't know the language or the culture. I had no authority here. I slumped down and lay against the warm earthen wall of their home. Large ants moved across my feet, burning them slightly as they bit me. Dragonflies lazed in the air currents. Inside I heard arguing in words I could only guess at. An hour passed.

Basilia came outside. "She is only two centimetres dilated. They let us examine her. That's a good start. The head is still high. They say she has no right to go to hospital, which they must decide. They have no money for the hospital fees or for transport. I said we can bring her. We can pay. Is that all right? We don't have much time."

We quickly explained we could bring this woman, her family, and the traditional birth attendant to the hospital. It was a difficult one-hour drive. It would have been an impossible journey of several hours on foot. Very few people in Upper West have vehicles. We arrived at the Tumu District Hospital. I got out and stormed in. I could speak English here. I asked for the doctor in charge. "We have a young woman with an obstructed labour. She probably needs a C-section." The first nurse I saw asked how much money she had. "We have no time. She needs care now. If she has no money, I'll pay."

"No, we cannot spoil them," I was told. "They have to know they need to pay."

I insisted that the young woman had to be helped, now!

It was another two hours of arguing before she was admitted. She was forced to lie on her back when she was struggling to labour, instead of squatting as she had at home. It was another hour before the theatre was ready and the nurse anaesthetist had been found, only slightly drunk, at her house adjacent to the hospital. By the time the Caesarean section was performed, the baby, a boy, was dead. A tear was already visible, the beginning of a vesico-vaginal fistula from her obstructed labour.

"You see!" her family shouted. "She has been punished. We have been punished. We should have let her die in the village. We have no grandson. And she is worthless to us without that boy. Now we are ashamed. Even though you have paid the money, what have we received? A dead child and a worthless woman!" Seething with rage and sorrow, they left to prepare to bury the dead baby, bring the teenage mother home, and begin the proceedings for their son to divorce her.

Shaking, I looked wordlessly at Basilia and Georgina. We said nothing to one another as we carried out our routine visit to this district hospital, poring over the immunization records and comparing the prenatal visits with the attended deliveries, now understanding why so few women delivered in the hospitals or clinics.

Later I told Basilia and Georgina about the woman we had tried to help on our way to the region, offering her a lift, only to have her husband take it in her stead and threaten to beat her if we tried to intercede. They shrugged. "What can we do? We try to fight for the women here, but we know how hard it is for them to get money to help them care for their children, to get permission to travel to take these sick children to health clinics, to understand simple directions to care for infections such as pneumonia or conditions like diarrhea and dehydration. We know when women get a little money they use it for school fees for their children or food and medicines for their family. When men get money, they drink, they buy women, and they beat their wives. What are we to do? At least you are here to encourage us."

It seemed it was slower here for changes to take place with women. In Bangladesh they were starting to travel independently from men. This had been encouraged by women working in the garment industry. Women had more economic power, and half of them used family planning so they could control fertility. These two facts, money and the ability to control their fertility, could help women change faster.

The status of women in Upper West was so low that they could be sold into marriage for a few cows and then be required to do most of the heavy labour. Despite Catholic mission hospitals providing good care for pregnant women, it wasn't surprising that the region's death rates for infants and children under five were the highest in Ghana, much of this because of high deaths in newborns reflecting the poor maternal health care.[8] It is important to distinguish newborn deaths (under one month because of poor delivery care), which is a component of infant (under one year) and under-five mortality (under five years). Post-neonatal death (one month to one year) and under-five mortality can be brought down by dealing with infectious disease by immunization and treatment of malaria, pneumonia, and diarrhea, but neonatal deaths are the slowest to improve because maternal health is poor.

Family planning, which allows women to space births safely, is the most cost-effective way to save the lives of pregnant women and infants. The Catholic doctor in charge of the hospital in Jirapa understood this and was supportive when I took time away from his hospital to work outside its gates, where the Danish government was funding the Ghanaian government health service to provide a family planning clinic, something the diocese could tolerate at a safe distance.

I met Alima Idris, a largely self-taught nursing assistant who had some on-the-job training she had been able to acquire at the hospital. Bright and sparkling with intelligence, she was competent and careful. Alima ran the family planning clinic, though the medical superintendent of the hospital had plans for her if she could be upgraded. Unfortunately, the government of Ghana had changed the entry requirements for nurses, so Alima needed more secondary school courses in mathematics and physics. There was no way to credit her for the practical skills she had learned, and the girls in Upper West had lower levels of education than those in other parts of the country. This meant there were few nurses from that region who could be employed to work in the districts where they would speak the local languages and understand the customs.

Alima chatted with me as we discussed the patients we had seen. I asked her how she had come to be a nursing assistant.

"I needed to do something to keep myself after my husband threw me out. My parents wouldn't take me back. They had received cows for me. And they were ashamed of me, for I wasn't a good mother. I had left my children. I love my children. They would be starting secondary school. I miss them. I haven't seen them for six years. Their father has forbidden it.

I was beaten, and he threw me into the yard, bleeding. But he was right to do what he did. I had disagreed with him. I understand that if a wife is late with the dinner, or burns the food, or goes out without permission, or disobeys her husband, he must do this.[9] But I couldn't agree. Every night he would bring home a woman, or two women, and I would have to sleep on the floor while they took my place in his bed. I was frightened. I know about these sicknesses, like AIDS. I was afraid. He would beat me in front of the children, and I was ashamed. I couldn't please my husband."

Alima also took turns on the maternity ward in the hospital. Although the hospital was Catholic, many of the staff members were Muslim, and there were no religious tensions. Many of the patients, like Alima, had suffered circumcision or female genital cutting, which is widespread, though illegal. As we had witnessed in Sudan, the women who had been mutilated had more difficult labours, often tearing terribly. Alima remarked, "I know they are suffering, but they must be clean for their husbands." They saw women's natural genitals as a sign of dirtiness, of shame.

Dr. Banka was the medical superintendent at Jirapa. He and Dr. Appiah, the regional director of health in Upper West, had organized radio programs against female circumcision. They had also spoken out about other forms of violence against women. These doctors talked in different local dialects on the radio and wrote in several languages in the local paper to explain that a prolonged labour wasn't the result of a woman's infidelity.

I also worked in the regional hospital in Wa. The crowded obstetrics and gynecology wards were full of other cases of obstructed labour and ruptured uteruses. I understood better when one woman, Aisha, explained, "I was having trouble with the baby. It was my first. I knew I should deliver in my mother-in-law's home. But after two days the family started to beat me. I had to confess the name of the man I had committed adultery with. I had only been with my husband. They thought I was being punished by Allah with this difficult birth for my bad behaviour. It was only when I lost consciousness that they brought me to the hospital. But the baby had died, and they could not repair my womb, which had burst. They had to remove it. Now I will never have children." I had seen this before, but now I understood more clearly, since the last time had been filtered through translation.

The wards were understaffed and not very clean, and patients slept two to a bed. On the gynecology ward many of the patients were young teenage girls who had been admitted with septic abortion. Adolescent premarital sex was the norm; many girls started having children by the age of eighteen. Even though I worked with the Ghanaian government nurses for the next several years to get family planning established at the local government clinics, I discovered that teenagers didn't want to come. We tried a discreet clinic one day a week in the local library in Wa, in a private room, but still with no success and a lot of resistance from parents and the churches.

Betty was one patient who had been admitted in septic shock from an illegal abortion. "Our parents won't let us use birth control. The boys say we have to have sex with them and they don't like to use condoms. What could I do? If I fell pregnant, I would be expelled from school. I tried the only way out I could find. Now I am ruined. They had to take away my womb, it was so infected. At least I am alive. But I can never have children. I thought if I was with an older man he would be more careful. The father of my baby was my teacher at school. He said it would be safe."

Basilia, Georgina, and several other nurses in Upper West were taught to ride motorcycles, and conducted outreach clinics with confidence. No one laughed when they came blazing in, helmets on and big grins on their faces. Three of these excellent nurses became district medical officers. Few doctors came to Upper West, so we had fought to have nurses who came and stayed be given responsibility to lead health care in the districts.

Years after I first worked in Upper West, careful research in Ghana showed the many barriers to skilled attendants at delivery: the tragic mix of poverty, low status of women, lack of education for girls, religious and cultural barriers, and user fees. All of these combined to create three delays: keeping women from seeking care, from getting to care, and from receiving care once they arrived at a hospital. Donors, including Denmark and the United Nations, tried, on an experimental basis, to pay for maternity care for women in the three poorest regions in the country, including Upper West.[10]

The increase in supervised deliveries and emergency obstetric care convinced the Department for International Development in Britain to use its own budget to support the government of Ghana to pay for maternal health in the National Health Insurance Scheme.[11]

Still, death rates of pregnant women are too high in Ghana, and the country isn't on track to meet UN targets to improve this. In the poorest provinces progress is slow, and female genital mutilation remains a problem. About one-quarter of women in Ghana report being beaten, a statistic that is higher in the northern regions.[12]

At a meeting to address why maternal health was not on track, the government tried to ignore the issue that family planning was not covered in the national health insurance scheme, even though it is the most cost-effective intervention to save women's lives.[13]

But things are moving. Plans are underway to take a model piloted in Bangladesh to train community-based midwives who will deliver women in their own homes and communities, recognizing we need to combine the cultural values of the home and family with the skills and technology of medical care and intervention.[14]

Like the yellow taxi that Lise repaired by switching fuses, sometimes we are travelling in the dark, but at least we are moving.

GLOBAL REFLECTION, 2018

When Theresa in Papua New Guinea lamented that she did not have the freedom I had as a woman, she may not have realized that gender itself is a powerful unifier. Socio-economic status, race, and power differentials are modifiers. What brings these all into play? It's the dynamics of development.

Haiti, for example, has been in the news. Oxfam staff have been involved in a prostitution scandal. Earlier, also in Haiti, a couple of hundred UN peacekeepers were sent home after being caught using child prostitutes. None were punished. In South Sudan, to which I returned in 2015 as part of a team evaluating Canadian support of mother-and-child health, UN peacekeepers were also involved with child prostitutes. The UN Mission in South Sudan repatriated four Bangladeshi personnel for engaging with child prostitutes. The tragedy of UN peacekeepers sexually exploiting children in their care was first raised in 1996 by Graça Machel, the UN independent expert on the impact of armed conflict on children and former minister of education in Mozambique. She reported that 50 percent of countries studied showed an increase in child prostitution after the arrival of peacekeepers.

Over the next two decades, continued UN reports verified this persistent crime in Democratic Republic of Congo, Northern Mali, Liberia, South Sudan, and Haiti, among other countries. Few of these peacekeepers used condoms, so pregnancy and the spread of HIV added to the drastic consequences.[15]

Unfortunately, it is not only UN peacekeepers who have normalized gender-based violence and sexual exploitation. I was the team leader, and only woman, of a mission in the Philippines addressing health needs of the urban poor in 1991. A lavish dinner was held by a company that did business with the UN agencies and bilateral government development workers. Only men were invited, so my team went off to enjoy great food, alcohol, and the company of semi-naked Filipina women. All of the invited men were development workers. I was chastised for being too uptight when I criticized this behaviour.

A few years later I was working in Zambia. Here the exploitation was about power and race, not gender, but there was still intimate partner violence. A very senior manager in a very prestigious UN agency had been raping his male driver. The male driver had some supports from the HR department and tried to go on with his life and with his family. The principal executive and his family were transferred to another country, and someone came from the headquarters of the UN agency to do "damage control." I would talk to this UN investigator in the restaurant of the Intercontinental Hotel in Lusaka. I was, of course, not allowed into the bar. I was a woman. The only women allowed in the bar were Zambian prostitutes to service the expatriate male guests.

Following this, I was in Bangladesh with a challenging assignment to evaluate health service delivery as part of an annual review. I had worked in Bangladesh a couple of dozen times. At a typical "development gathering" — women in silk and rubies comparing house staff, and men talking tennis — a colleague became very drunk. He was angry I had not taken a job with the World Bank mission based in Dhaka. He started to shout at me and then grabbed my breast. When I removed his hand from my body, he slugged me in the head.

This was witnessed by the host, who thought it might be time to summon the various drivers and try to bring the party to a gracious close. Luckily, another colleague, who was also drunk, fell and broke some furniture, causing a distraction.

Now, I am from northern Ontario. Fending off a drunken male is actually a skill I developed from an early age. And my intention had been to ignore this. I had work to do, and I was not going to let this episode get in my way. The problem was, word got back to the leader of the Canadian delegation, my boss. I was given a lecture on gender-based violence and how there should be zero tolerance; more than 12 percent of maternal deaths in Bangladesh may stem from intimate partner violence. I had to go to the head of the World Bank mission in Dhaka, point out which breast and where I was slugged in the head, and then do the same with the Canadian Head of Aid and the Canadian High Commissioner. And what was the solution? I was told that in order to protest this behaviour, I had to go home — and not do the job Canada had sent me to do.

So I got a lesson in why people do not disclose sexual harassment. It's because, too often, the victim gets blamed. As it turned out, I refused to leave. I carried on with my job, and the World Bank perpetrator was never disciplined.

Another assignment, a decade later, in another country, for a different development agency. The married head of the regional office has his staff pimp women for him, lovely Southeast Asian beauties. His staff feel unable to protest. He is the boss.

In Papua New Guinea, where I have worked extensively, women face at least a 50 percent lifetime risk of rape.[16,17] Workers at a Canadian-owned mine were found to be raping women: a Human Rights Watch report, *Gold's Costly Dividend: Human Rights Impacts of Papua New Guinea's Porgera Gold Mine*, "identifies systemic failures on the part of Toronto-based Barrick Gold that kept the company from recognizing the risk of abuses, and responding to allegations that abuses had occurred. The report examines the impact of Canada's failure to regulate the overseas activities of its companies and also calls on Barrick to address environmental and health concerns around the mine with greater transparency.

> "We interviewed women who described brutal gang rapes by security guards at Barrick's mine," said Chris Albin-Lackey, senior business and human rights researcher at Human Rights Watch. "The company should have acted long before Human Rights Watch conducted its research and prompted them into action."[18]

It is deeply troubling when powerful, wealthier men condone sexual harassment, exploitation, and violence against women and men and children, and this means we have a real problem in the development business that undermines our good intentions. Somehow, this has to be addressed in a way that changes culture, stops normalizing this behaviour, and does not punish the victims. But the gender, power, and money relationships can work both ways, either way driving the HIV epidemic.

Sub-Saharan Africa is the worst region in the world for HIV. The Caribbean is second. The following are memories from my travels to both regions.

He's a white South African — balding, grey-haired, with a considerable paunch — wearing sandals, a safari shirt, and shorts. Maybe age fifty-five? She is looking a little bored, in a very bright, shiny, low-cut lilac blouse, skin-tight jeans, and blue open-toed platform heels. The Club beer in her hand is emptying slowly as she alternates sips with languid drags on her cigarette. They don't speak much to one another.

I try not to meet her eyes. I had met Grace yesterday, but today she is at work. Yesterday, she was explaining why she does this work. She is twenty, and her four-year-old daughter is playing in the hotel pool under the care of Grace's friend and co-worker.

Grace was forced to leave school in the Upper West Region, in Ghana, when she became pregnant. She had no funds to continue her schooling or to support herself or her child. Her family was embarrassed by the pregnancy, the father of the baby unwilling to help. Grace finishes her beer. Her client pulls her to her feet and propels her back into the hotel.

Yesterday Grace explained how she had started in the Upper West Region, which continues to be one of the poorest regions in Ghana in spite of the economic development that is quickly moving the country to middle-income status. There, women average six children, assume violence against them is justified, and begin child-bearing as teenagers. There, Grace earned less for a night of work than the price of a few beers. There, the police would raid the house where she worked and demand sex instead of jail. She explained how she moved on to a gold-mining area where she and her friends would hire a truck to visit the mines and make more in one night than they could make in a month farther north. She lived in Kumasi before coming here. And she is now earning good money in Accra. Here, she insists on condoms with her clients but not with her boyfriends.

Grace knows that 30–75 percent of women who do sex work are HIV positive but is afraid to be tested for HIV.

Sue is a little bitter. Forty years old, a Canadian, her marriage faltered to a halt three months earlier after fifteen years and two children. "Take a break," her teaching friends tell her. "Go heal your wounds. Get some sun."

Two weeks in the tanning bed, highlights in her hair, five pounds of weight finally lost. Three new bathing suits. Seductive sarongs.

She arrives in Tobago. The shade of blue in the water astounds her. The lazy grace of the people, their lilt, that accent she cannot quite fully decipher. By day two she has braids and beads in her hair, and has caught the eye of Wesley, who teaches snorkelling. She cannot believe her luck. He is gorgeous! The tight black curls of his hair, his deep brown eyes, the mahogany skin of his well-muscled limbs. How his eyes light up when he sees her. She's forty years old and he must be half her age. Go cougar!

By day three they take all of their meals together. Naturally, she buys his drinks. It is an easy evolution that he join her discreetly in her bed, in the fan-cooled villa, with the sound of the waves outside the white wooden-shuttered windows. She is honoured to help his family with the new roof for their house and to leave money behind for his sister's school fees when she tearfully boards her morning plane to return to Canada. She will write. She will come back. Her beach boy will await her.

By four in the afternoon, Wesley is meeting a new group of guests, and he catches the eye of a brunette, looking lonely.

We are all part of the development dance. We are in the midst of gender, power, money, and race relationships. Wittingly or innocently, we perpetuate transactions. There is a casting couch of development, scholarships, and jobs offered to women of colour in exchange for sexual favours provided to well-known international development jet setters. Human beings are vulnerable away from their homes and families. Pretending that this is not so, that it does not happen to us, blinds us to our role in these development contracts. I remember speaking with one friend who had been working in a conflict zone. She laughed. At the various interagency meetings, she would look around the room and realize she had slept with every man there. "At least I wasn't sleeping with the locals, like the men!"

One Day My Child Was Playing, the Next Day He Had Died:

Bangladesh, Ghana, Ethiopia, and Nigeria

Bangladesh, 1993

Poor countries such as Bangladesh can save the lives of children under five years of age by bringing simple low-cost interventions to poor people. Immunizing children can save lives from diseases such as tetanus and measles. Teaching mothers to watch for signs of pneumonia, get antibiotics for their children, and make sugar and salt solutions or other oral rehydration drinks for diarrhea can save the lives of children from those infections. NGOs, outreach health workers, and community-level education can reduce the deaths of children under five by at least one-third without investing in expensive hospital-level care.

Chattering children ran to see us, excited by the presence of a foreigner. They laughingly followed the health worker and me as we took a little path through the rice paddies and fish ponds. White cattle egrets soared overhead, and roosters scratched in the sand outside. We entered a courtyard where a few women in gently flowing cotton saris laid out lentils on the ground.

Inside a small round house made of branches plastered with cow dung and mud, two veiled women in the dark room greeted us with shy smiles. Chandra and Rajani were sisters. Chandra was the elder — at nineteen, already the proud mother of a two-year-old son, Mizan. Mizan had diarrhea, and Chandra was preparing an oral rehydration drink for him. She had boiled water, which was cooling in a pan on the wood fire, and had washed her hands in a basin with soap.

Carefully, Chandra used a cup to ladle out five cups of water into a jug, counting as she went. "Ek, dui, tin [theen], char, pa[n]ch." Four bangles clicked and clanged at her wrist as she pinched salt from a small dish in her fingers to approximate one-half level teaspoon. "Ek!" she said proudly, scooping up a handful of sugar from a little sack. "Chhoi." She was explaining that this was the equivalent of six level teaspoons.[1]

Chandra stirred the mixture and mashed in a little banana, feeding her son with a spoon until he drank about a half cup. She then coaxed him back onto her breast. "I also feed him green coconut water," she said, through the health worker. "I have learned this and many more things. For six months I only gave breast milk. Then I added mashed vegetables and fish, dahl, banana. I bring him to be weighed and measured with the health worker to see if he is growing well, at the same time as he gets his needles and vitamin A. We are happy that the health worker comes to deliver our babies. Now we feel safer."

I had returned to Bangladesh in 1993 as the team leader of a child survival project concerning urban slums and poor rural communities for World Vision, a humanitarian organization dedicated to helping children and addressing the root causes of poverty. Anjali, the health worker from the project, was accompanying me.

Anjali and I thanked the women for their time and climbed back into our rickshaw, brightly coloured with movie star faces, shiny metal ornaments, health messages, and the logo of the project. We travelled slowly on slightly squeaking wheels toward a different kind of poverty — a rank, sewage-filled corner of the city of Chittagong. The stench and heat assaulted us as we reached a makeshift hovel with a torn cloth acting as an entrance.

Anjali carried a bag with a stethoscope, a blood pressure cuff, a measuring tape, and a thermometer. We lifted the curtain at the doorway and called out a greeting in Bangla. One room was home to three generations. Alamgir was twenty-four and worked as a rickshaw *wallah*. His widowed mother, wife, and six-month-old son lived with him. Alamgir, who was home today for our visit, explained what his family had learned from the project. "My son was sick. Anjali has taught us well. When he got sick, he was coughing. We borrowed a watch and counted his breathing. It was sixty times a minute![2] His chest muscles were pulling in. We knew he had pneumonia and were able to bring him to the clinic for antibiotics. He is improving well."

According to Anjali, the Chittagong project had exceeded the goals it had hoped to accomplish by 1996, ahead of schedule, for improved nutrition and safe drinking water. Babies no longer got tetanus as newborns, birth attendants had been trained to do cleaner deliveries, and mothers were immunized against tetanus when they were pregnant. The project had nearly reached its final goals for immunization, vitamin A distribution, and oral rehydration therapy and would easily meet them in the three years left in the project. Breastfeeding was being promoted, and the project was finding better ways to teach mothers to recognize when their children had pneumonia, such as using small manual counters to measure rapid breaths, since few had watches or knew their numbers.

As women received more education, they were better able to watch for sicknesses and manage them to save their children's lives.[3] But still, boys were given better care and food when they were ill than girls. A small boy was more likely to be brought to a clinic when he was sick than his sister. This would take much longer to change. Boys under one year are weaker biologically than girls, and death rates are higher for boys in that age group. But as the children get older, the girls receive much less care, so by the time they are five, the death rates are higher for girls.[4]

There have been some important changes. As of 2012, the under-five mortality rate is higher in Bangladesh for males than females (44:38 per 1,000 live births), suggesting that girls are now increasingly, appropriately, brought to care.[5]

Back at the project office I studied the files. In the adjacent clinic I watched the way children were cared for and interviewed the health workers and community development workers. I said my farewells to the project staff in Chittagong and praised their hard work, then began a long journey by rickshaw, boat, car, and plane back to Dhaka.

In 1993 Dhaka had eight million people, with a slum population of more than three million. Hundreds of thousands of people lived on the streets in makeshift shelters with plastic sheeting overhead.[6] Home, located alongside a railway embankment, might be a tiny patch surrounding a small cookstove. Another family would live close by and beside them another.

There were about 200,000 street children living in Dhaka then. Estimates now vary from 333,000 street children in Dhaka to 450,000. Some were forced into prostitution; others picked rags, chipped bricks, or sold flowers to make a few taka a day for food and lodging. The impressive drops in the death rates of children under five in Bangladesh, declines of over 4 percent per year, hadn't been seen in street children. Increasing urbanization had brought more children to live in urban streets, and this group had extremely limited access to health care.[7]

Through the translator, I spoke with a young girl named Mallika, crouching so that I was at her level as she stood solemnly in a tattered and faded yellow dress over ragged blue-and-yellow trousers. She seemed about eight years old and was painfully thin with bony wrists, but her luminous brown eyes lit up when she talked.

"It was better when I could work in the factory with my mother. I could earn a few taka. But now there are new rules. Children aren't allowed to work there. I am supposed to go to school instead. We don't have the money to pay for school. There is just my mother and me. I never knew my father. There is no one to look after me during the day. I am alone now. I do what I can. I don't earn as much. The police chase me and beat me sometimes if they catch me begging on the street. But I am pretty, they say. If I let them touch me, they leave me alone." She pointed shyly to her tiny breast buds, which dimpled her dress, and gestured vaguely to her pubic area, hidden by her *shalwar kameez*. "I liked it better working with my mother; I could wind the thread and run errands and make money. Miss, do you know why they made the new rules?"

I shook my head, unsure how I could explain that banning child labour was supposed to help her, not hurt her further, or whether I believed it, now that I was beginning to understand that for many children it was the best of several bad choices.

The day before I was scheduled to leave Bangladesh was the day a general strike, or *hartal,* was planned. These are frightening events of organized chaos. I had experienced them before, including during my first visit to Bangladesh. I wasn't looking forward to living through another one; already my heart had begun to beat a little faster. After long days of writing my conclusions, I was overwhelmed by the needs of the people here. I couldn't solve the problems, but I could at least finish my report showing the strong progress in the project and hope for continued funding.

I hopped into a baby taxi to go to the project office to leave a hard copy and an electronic version of the report. When that was completed, I felt emotionally exhausted. The project staff suggested I not make the forty-five-minute trip to my guest house alone in case there was trouble in the streets. "Nonsense!" I retorted. "I was here when the government fell. I had to be taken to the airport by ambulance, since they were the only vehicles allowed to travel because of the violence. I'll be fine today." I left the office by baby taxi, which took me about halfway home, then was stopped in the middle of a riot in which the police were keeping order with clubs. People ran from the uniformed police, screaming. Soldiers smashed at the baby taxis and bent their metal fenders. My driver grabbed the taka notes I had in my hand, pushed me out of the vehicle, and sped off down a side street, grinding gears.

A woman who had also gotten out of her baby taxi led me quickly along the street. She talked to me in Bangla, perhaps explaining what was happening. I gathered that the opposition party was enforcing the *hartel* and had ordered all motorized vehicles to stop. Rickshaws on the road were picking up stranded travellers. My guide led me by the arm and found a rickshaw for me. I got in, passed hand to hand by Bangladeshi passersby. The hood on the rickshaw was put down to hide my head, and I was relieved that I was wearing a *shalwar kameez.* No foreigners were evident that day; only local people were out. Expatriates with our obvious wealth could be targeted for robbery and attack in the violence that was surging throughout the city. Before I could thank my Muslim Samaritan, the rickshaw *wallah* started to pedal with his sandal-clad feet, his *lungi* loosely wrapped around his waist, his calf muscles straining.

I couldn't communicate with the rickshaw *wallah* who seemed to have been given general instructions by my benefactress. There were police and shouting crowds, and my rapidly beating heart firmly announced to my terrified mind that I was frightened. Nonsense … I'll be fine. Had I said that? Who was I kidding! Despite being covered, my white woman's skin made me feel so exposed. We kept moving, stopping several times to ask storekeepers, "English?" If they nodded, I showed them the address I was trying to reach.

As the comforting sounds of the driver pedalling the rickshaw brought me closer to my guest house, I thought about my mother. She combined her work as a journalist/politician/social worker/community organizer with homemade jams and jellies and great comfort food. The strain of the multiple roles made her always a little anxious. She had told me I shouldn't make this trip because of the danger. She should talk! As a journalist, she was on the last plane out of Cuba during the Missile Crisis. As a role model, she helped create the life I led. She was the one who had sent me a cartoon clipping saying, "Any idiot can handle a crisis. It's day-to-day living that gets you down."

I thought about my daughter, who once wrote in a class assignment: "I was afraid when my mother was in Bangladesh and we heard frightening things about the government falling."

The sounds of the rioting receded as we neared Gulshan, a quiet, leafy suburb of embassies and expatriate houses. After another thirty minutes, I arrived at my own safe guest house, alighted from the rickshaw, paid the driver, and went inside.

A few hours after the excitement of the *hartal*, I met several old friends for dinner. I looked around the table. We were dressed in smooth silk and drank alcohol — forbidden in Bangladesh except in selected foreigners' enclaves and homes — and talked about tennis. None of us had servants at home; none of us would wear silk for such a casual get-together. Even in Dhaka we remained untouched by the fighting still raging outside.

After dinner I was brought home not by baby taxi but by a prearranged driver, who chose streets that were far from the ongoing fighting. I arrived again at my guest house and stepped out of the vehicle, eyes carefully averted from the scattered street children selling roses. I had done my report; I hoped that somehow it would help these children. A very small girl in a tattered *shalwar kameez* thrust a handful of red sweet-smelling flowers toward me. In careful English she stammered, "Miss ... for you ... no money." Her grubby hand had enfolded my white ringed hand in hers, giving me a single perfect rose.

This beautiful Bangladeshi child was surviving. She was living ... and giving.

First Mission, Ghana, 1994

After the mission in Bangladesh, I returned to Ghana's Upper West to work with Jens, helping the regional health authorities to strengthen primary health care, particularly for children and pregnant women. From 1992 to 1996, Jens worked in Ghana for the Danish government (for Danida, the Danish International Development Agency) as the technical team leader for its health projects. He had asked me to come onboard, and before long I found myself spending one month at a time, three times a year, in Ghana.

The death rate of infants and children under five was about 25 percent higher in rural Ghana than in the country's urban areas, and the number of children's deaths in Ghana was greater than in Bangladesh.[8] Larger distances between villages in the rural areas of Ghana made it harder to get outreach workers to conduct immunization and other child survival strategies. The number of deaths of pregnant women was higher in Ghana, too, due to the lack of family planning and higher fertility and high-risk pregnancy. If deaths of pregnant women were high in numbers, so were the number of deaths of their newborns, reflecting the lack of good obstetric care.[9]

Abigail, a Ghanaian public health nurse, and I made the long but now familiar journey from Accra, Ghana's capital, to Wa. Chatting on the way about our lives and the stress of juggling work and family, we smiled at each other as we passed trucks that bore hopeful sayings: BY HIS GRACE, FEAR NOT, GLORIOUS TOUCH. It was a tiring eighteen hours before we arrived in Wa and unpacked our belongings in the guest house.

The next day we met with the Regional Health Management Team, including my friends, the capable nurses Basilia and Georgina. Our first

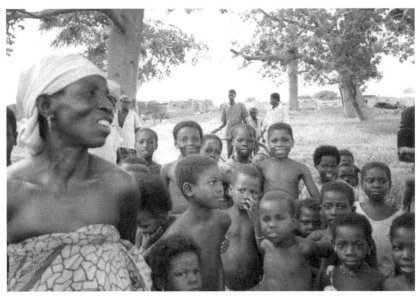

Women and children in Ghana's Upper West Region prepare to be immunized.

order of business was to immunize communities against yellow fever and cerebrospinal meningitis. As I had learned when working in northern Ontario's Indigenous communities, health workers must first show respect to the local chief before starting any health activities. We began the morning meeting in the chief's palace (a larger version of the villagers' homes made of mud, straw, and cow dung). In return he sat and supported us for the entire day as we immunized children among the huge crowds of people surging about and arguing. Afterward the chief presented us with yams and a live guinea fowl for our dinner, and we drank *pitoh*, the foamy, slightly sweet and sour millet or guinea corn beer.

By 1994 we knew the region well from our challenging struggle to improve mother-and-child health services but continued to find the work difficult, with little progress achieved. Abigail and I visited the clinics, sometimes finding no nurses there (salaries didn't come for months, so the nurses had to work on their family farms for food). Often we found the nurse in charge drunk, lonely, and discouraged. The clinics seldom had enough medicines, and to offset missing salaries, nurses resorted to charging patients illegally in order to have money to live on.

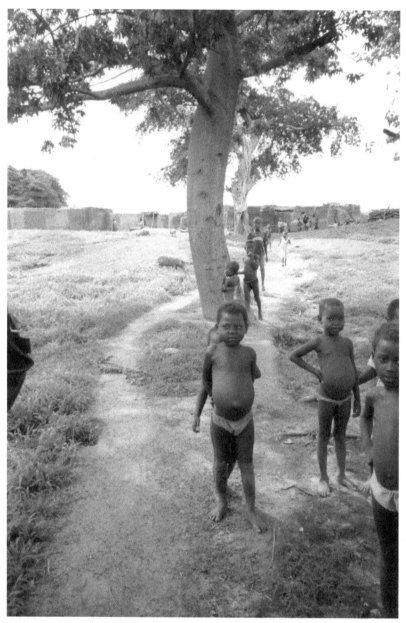

Malnourished children gather in Upper West, Ghana.

In another village we, along with a couple of feisty Ghanaian nurses, did growth monitoring to detect malnutrition and to arrange extra feeding for the many babies who were simply starving. Some babies got weighed, but very few, because of the lack of staff. One of the nurses seemed cruelly indifferent when a mother brought in a terribly malnourished child, but I realize now that she knew how soon that child would die, how quickly that small life would end. Malnourished children are much more likely to die — poverty, hunger, infectious disease, and death spiral viciously.[10]

In a village near Tumu we listened to Frannie, a nurse who was frustrated about the hungry children she was trying to help in the hospital. "Look at this boy! Look how thin he is — four years old with this hugely swollen belly! His mother is trying to carry on with five children, no money, and she is pregnant again. The father was here yesterday visiting from the gold mine where he works near Kumasi. He wore an expensive bright shirt and a new watch but left no money to help feed that child and hurriedly went back to the mine." Frannie was bitter and told me a bad joke I'd heard before. "How do you tell a community that has food aid? The men have new watches."

I thought to myself, sadly, that much of the miner husbands' money went to pay sex workers, helping HIV to escalate out of control.

Friendships formed quickly in Ghana, just as plants placed in Ghana's hot, moist red earth grew fast and furiously. Whenever we felt discouraged by the slow progress, we were buoyed by people's warmth. There was Abu, who ran the Uplands Hotel in Wa with his illiterate father. He always had a smile for us, always encouraged us, saying our work was important. And there was Lydia, Abigail's cousin, who lent me her murder mysteries. And there was my little friend, ten-year-old Evelyn, whom I had met while I was collecting brightly coloured stones for my children. She was the smartest in her local Catholic school, with a bright future ahead of her.

While visiting small communities throughout Upper West, we stopped to see one of the oldest mosques in West Africa. A near riot ensued in the village as children begged for pens or pencils for school. We gave them all we had, but it wasn't nearly enough for everyone. The kids cried and fought among themselves. Had our presence in the village made things better or worse? We left feeling guilty.

In early 1994 we had been working in Upper West for nearly a month and had only a few days left before returning to Accra. A fax from Jens, who was based mostly in the capital overseeing several linked projects, arrived in the regional government office and was brought over to the health directorate. "Do not return by road," the message said. "Wait for a military plane to evacuate you next weekend. There is trouble to the south."

Normally, there was little news on the radio. When Abigail and I tuned in, we heard only ambiguous information. There was mention of a "disturbance" in the Tamale area in Northern Region that had been contained.

We asked around if anyone had received any more news, for example, from their relatives to the south of us. Northern Region is actually south of Upper West, which is on the northern border of Ghana and Burkina Faso. No one had heard anything. And then convoys of white evacuees started to arrive — priests and construction teams.

Jens's directive had been triggered by the fact that in Northern Region, disagreement between the Dagombas and the Kokombas over the ownership of a guinea fowl had turned into such violent ethnic fighting that six hundred were now dead, a number that quickly escalated into the thousands.[11] Seven children were slaughtered the day before we received our fax, and there were heads on spikes in the town of Tamale, which was several hours south by road. Pregnant women had been disembowelled, fetuses cut out of their bodies.

In the bar at the Uplands Hotel we found out more details. Father Declan, from the White Fathers order, had just arrived and told us that the Catholic churches were burning. The churches had sheltered fleeing pregnant women and children from both sides in this bitter tribal conflict. This wasn't acceptable, so the churches were set on fire. The schools were closed, and the seminarians had fled from the south northward to safer towns such as Wa. An anthropologist who was also sitting in the bar and slowly drinking a Club beer was smug about everything, saying it served the "goddamn churches" right, a strangely bitter comment. She was slightly drunk, and I chose not to question her about the comment, fearing it would only intensify her hostility.

Later, over dinner, I talked with Father Declan, who had devoted his life to helping Africans and was struggling to understand the tribal fighting that had caused so much suffering and death. He had lived in Ghana, based in Tamale, for twenty-five years and had narrowly avoided death himself, screeching past the checkpoints on the road.

Father Declan was hungry for literary conversation and cultural connection. By our second beer, we were talking about writing and our favourite authors. He asked me about William Faulkner. What did I think of his acceptance speech for the Nobel Prize?[12] I hadn't read it? "[Man] is immortal ... because he has a soul, a spirit capable of compassion and sacrifice and endurance." Had I read Graham Greene? Did I know he had been a spy in Sierra Leone?[13] Did I think it was right that his books were put on a prohibited list of ones that Catholics shouldn't read? And what about Brian Moore? Did I think these two — Greene and Moore — were Catholic writers or writers who were Catholic?

This was heady stuff as we sat under the mango trees and drank beer. Looking across at my clean-shaven, neatly dressed companion with his clerical collar and cool tropical clothing, I was reassured that some clergymen were highly literate and reasoned. He was smart and articulate, and his years of dedicated service showed that he was also a man of faith, a good man, a priest who was in trouble simply because he had driven a Kokomba mother and child to safety in the night in the midst of the conflict.

Father Declan had to leave the Tamale area because he had appeared to take sides in the fighting, but he was now safe in Wa. He worried, however, that there was no one left at the parish to give stirring talks about trying to uphold the dignity of African women, who did most of the work, or to organize small loans for them so they could better care for their children, to protect them from being beaten by their husbands, and to teach them to read. In every village the men seemed to sit around under trees, drinking. Without the need to watch cows and goats that their nomadic pastoralist society once required, life barely gave them a walk-on role. The women, however, still had their identity, still carried water and firewood, still cared for their children. They farmed and took care of everyone around them.

This White Father I had met had made me think, so I asked him, "Is it compassion and sacrifice that keeps bringing me here? Is it worth the risk to my own safety? I find myself asking these same questions in each place I visit. What am I doing here? What have I done that's worthwhile? What have I really achieved since I arrived? Will my fate be decided according to how I've lived out my life? Is this life like the dead reckoning on a sailing ship, plotting out our course based on where we were last and how we've moved to get here? Even animals move on their migrations this way. How do I measure my days? Not with T.S. Eliot's coffee spoons, but these one-month portions I give to different countries, searching for myself. Complicating the order of things with my new ideas, my affluence. Changing and being changed."

I felt so sad, so confused. Even as a seldom-practising Catholic, I wanted Father Declan's reassurance. "What have I done here?" I continued. "I've drunk *pitoh* and bought a kerosene lantern for Mavis, a traditional birth attendant, who was sobbing at the lack of light for night deliveries, so one newborn had died because she couldn't see the dark staining of meconium [fetal bowel movement] on the baby's head as it delivered, signalling fetal distress and requiring urgent intervention to deliver the baby more quickly. Is just being here and sharing all of this — witnessing — a contribution? Somewhere I have another life, a family who know nothing of this. How can I explain this life of mine to them? How can I share with my children this other world of poor children that keeps drawing me away from my own? How do you keep on working in this poor part of Ghana with so little progress? Do you really believe in God?"

Father Declan smiled and sipped his beer. "You're just tired. You've run out of faith. You have to keep on. Are you crazy? Why would I be doing this, living in the bush for twenty-five years, if I didn't believe in God?"

When I protested about the many dedicated people I had met in Africa who were humanitarian but not motivated by faith, he simply laughed. "To work under these conditions without faith, why that, too, is a faith!"

As the night sky sparkled overhead, he came close to convincing me there really was a loving God, a God who would encourage such a man to devote his life to serving the vulnerable, to show them they weren't forgotten. A God who could use this tragic conflict to bring intellectual stimulation to a hard-working priest.

The tribal fighting in northern Ghana was altering my life, as well.

Our health team was on the move. We had decided to ignore Jen's advice and take advantage of the protection afforded by a convoy of trucks containing construction workers. We had met the men — tanned English and Irish "old Africa hands" evacuated from Ghana's Northern Region — in the bar of the Uplands Hotel. They had sat at the next table to Father Declan and me, swapping stories over bottles of chilled Star and Club beer. The men had told us they were planning to return, hoping the fighting had settled down.

Abigail was expecting her fifth child and was anxious to see her husband and children. She had been away from them for two years while she studied for a master's degree in public health in the United States, and she had returned just a few months earlier. Almost immediately she had become pregnant. The family lived in Kumasi, which was reachable only by road.

As I packed to leave Wa, I happily recalled going to Mass at the local Catholic boys' school and hearing the children's beautiful voices soar in harmony. But to the south, churches were burning. It was heartbreaking that people were being stopped on the road to Kumasi and shot simply because they were Kokombas. We tried not to appear frightened.

We were set to leave at dawn. It wasn't yet the steaming heat of the tropics. The regional director of health services came to say goodbye and assured us that God wouldn't allow "a hair on your head to be harmed." It was time to pull up the connections I'd made here. Abu gave me mangoes and told me he would pray to Allah to keep us safe. I was grateful for Abu's friendship. He'd kept me afloat in difficult times. I gave him a hug and told him I'd be back soon. This place had started to feel like home. I felt completely torn up with loss and could hardly face leaving. I was also frightened of journeying through hours of tribal fighting.

Abu waved goodbye, both hands upraised. Abigail said a Christian prayer aloud, asking that we make it safely. "We are worried because we have heard such bad stories," she explained to God. Our driver Dominic, Abigail, and I all said "Amen." Then we set off on our journey, the two trucks from the construction company twenty minutes behind us.

It was a seven-hour trip to the first stop in Kumasi, where we intended to break the journey and stay with Abigail's family. The road was rough and slow going. Due to the constant clearing of the tropical rainforest, only a few sparse trees dotted the red soil. The arid day got hotter with every mile, but we were cooled by the erratic air conditioning that luckily was working that day. Ironically, the convoy of two road crew vehicles, which was our safety net and the reason we had decided to risk travelling by car, had disappeared from view. Somehow we had become separated from them, and now we could see no one on the road in either direction. We were aware we were on our own and drove for miles on empty roads accompanied only by a mix of fear and faith for the next four hours.

Suddenly, twenty or more armed men waved us to a stop. Some carried rusty old Kalashnikovs and others held knives, dusty spears, and pipes that blew darts poisoned with snake venom. There were a few boys among them, probably no older than twelve, and the rest were in their late teens. Some were as old as thirty. Dressed in rough, ragged clothes, they were nevertheless colourful, wearing shirts of brightly printed cotton or handwoven embroidery. Crocheted caps hugged their closely cropped heads. We didn't know if they were Dagombas or Kokombas.

Nervously we halted. I rolled down my window in the back seat, smiled, and said, "Good morning!" I was getting used to meeting people who rarely saw *nasalas*, or whites. People would come up to me and say, "Good morning, *nasala*!" And I would reply "Good morning!" and shake hands. So I reached through the window with a huge smile and started shaking their dry, rough hands with as much flourish as I could, with the snap and clasp of the ritualized handshakes of the region.

On cue they replied with big grins on their faces, "Good morning, *nasala*!"

The men gathered round the vehicle, and one of them pointed inside. He was so near that I smelled his strong sweat. I assumed he wanted water, so I passed him the bottle beside me. He shook his head and pointed again, this time miming he was taking a picture. I picked up the camera beside me with an inquisitive look. Big grin and a nod. Twelve men posed, guns pointed straight at us, and smiled. I took a picture. Other men rushed over from the side of the road, proud and eager to be in the next shot. I took it. They nodded cheerfully. And then we were done. We were through the barricade.

I was still shivering with the effort of the performance when Abigail said, "Praise the Lord!" Then we were back on the open road.

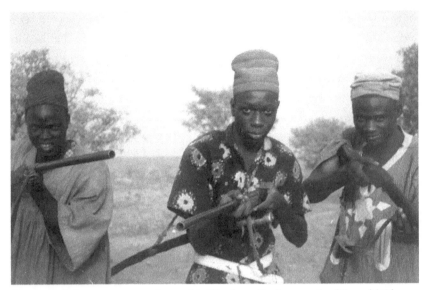

Dogomba fighters stop us on the road in Northern Region, north of Tamale, Ghana.

As I watched Abigail and Dominic continue to pray in thanksgiving, I was still shaking. But somehow it wasn't simple fear and relief we were feeling. There was also a sense of triumph. We had done it! We had gotten through! We felt we could cope with whatever came next. Whether it was God who travelled with us, or our own mix of skills and courage, we had what we needed for the journey.

SECOND MISSION, GHANA, 1994

I wanted to share with my family the spiritual epiphany I'd had in Ghana. Two months after the Guinea fowl war, I brought my eleven-year-old son, Alec, to Ghana. Jens had asked me to spend another month in Upper West, and I couldn't bear to leave my children yet again. So Jens simply said, "Bring Alec." The younger of my two children, he seemed the more vulnerable to my frequent absences.

Alec delighted in our few days in Accra, collecting rocks on the beach that had tumbled from the sand and waves, finding pieces of soft mica. He was excited to use his own French in the market, bargaining to buy a

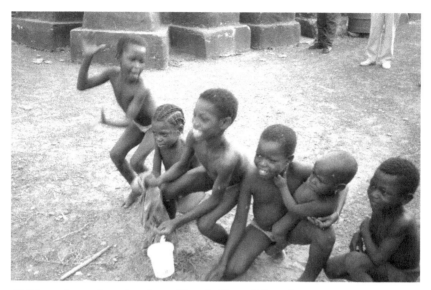

Children play and greet us in a village in Upper West, Ghana.

leather-wrapped knife from a Tuareg trader from Mali and talking with Jens's cook, Laurent, who was from Togo. Alec loved the taxis and trucks with their slogans of encouragement: DON'T GIVE UP, TRUST IN GOD, ALL SHALL PASS, SLOW BUT SURE.

We then continued north with Jens to Wa. Alec enjoyed the long, bumpy, red and dusty road, listening to Frank Sinatra (Jens's favourite) or gospel music (when the drivers picked the music). When we stopped in Kumasi at a local watering hole, Alec kicked a ball around with some kids he had just met. "The children here are so lucky," he told me. "They all dance when they greet us and seem so happy!"

When we arrived back at the Uplands Hotel, Abu greeted us. "Aleczi, you are coming with me and I am buying you a Coke. And I have some friends for you to meet. This is Abdulai, and this is Chris. We will teach you Dagaare and Wala."

A few hours later, exhausted, Alec went to bed. Abu came to greet me again after I had made sure Alec was sleeping well. He was happy to meet Alec. Abu proudly told me Alec wasn't "like a white boy — he doesn't act as if he finds us different from himself."

The next day Abu taught Alec a game played in the sand, which involved moving stones around carefully drawn diagonal lines. In return Alec taught Abu tic-tac-toe and showed him how to use a Game Boy.

Abu and Alec shared their lunch of roasted goat meat, which was brought to them by the cook. Alec was delighted that he had to use his hands to eat to be polite. They went to town together, Alec complaining with a huge grin that Abu was spoiling him. "He bought me a big jug of Coke and a handkerchief," he told me.

The next morning at 6:00 a.m. my little friend Evelyn came by. Alec was amazed that "morning" started so early, just after the sun rose. We arranged to invite Evelyn for dinner at the Uplands Hotel, then walked her home and played board games with her family. After that we drove into town to phone Alec's dad for his birthday, a complex and time-consuming challenge that took an hour and a half from the switchboard at the post office.

Each day brought new adventures. Alec found lizards, frogs, and a turtle bigger than his hand. He could answer longer and longer questions in Dagaare and spoke the language with the guards, who taught him a new game, different from the one he had learned from Abu. We went to Mass at the Xavier Boys' School, where Alec loved hearing the boys' choir sing in harmony to xylophones made of wood and drums.

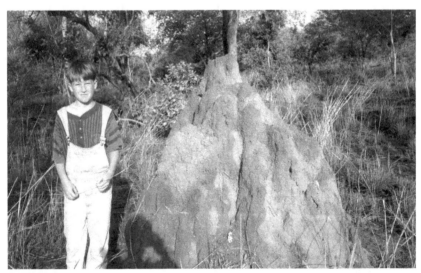

Alec Morrison, the author's son, beside an anthill in Upper West, Ghana.

After three days, and with Alec fully recovered from his jet lag, it was time to go farther afield. We visited a number of villages that had recently initiated some community development and primary health-care activities, including immunizing children, teaching mothers to prepare sugar and salt water rehydration drinks for diarrhea, and showing these same mothers how to recognize the warning signs of pneumonia, such as rapid breathing.

We drove north toward the Burkina Faso border. On the way we stopped to visit traditional bonesetters, who mended fractured hips, legs, and multiple traumas from road traffic accidents using homemade splints, casts, and traditional massage techniques. Some patients combined the strengths of two worlds, stopping first at the hospital for an X-ray, which they then brought to a traditional healer. In Tumu, this part of Upper West, bonesetters had been in one family for generations. All the male members were destined for this vocation and were taught it throughout their lives. Payment for their excellent care, regardless of the length of the treatment, was one black fowl and a calabash filled with white cowrie shells. The former was easier to obtain and payable at the first presentation, the latter after successful treatment.

Satisfied patients seemed much happier in this environment than in the "modern," under-equipped hospital where payment was in cash. In the bonesetters' family compound, the family could also stay with the patient, helping to prepare meals. Many of the patients were children who had fallen out of fruit trees, breaking their legs, often called "mango fractures." The rooms were individual mud huts made the same way as village homes. The bonesetters understood that people had no money, so patients could barter yams to pay for herbal medicines that were rubbed into skin to promote healing of underlying bones.

The local tale that the eldest bonesetter, Kwadwo, told us proudly was that "our special gifts of healing can only occur in our own place, as the spirits who have given these gifts reside here." He told us that one of their great-grandmothers past had been given this gift after a fight with a rival wife in their polygamous society. She had broken the pounding mortar of her rival, and the break had been miraculously healed, so this family now had the gift to heal broken bones like the mortar of the legend. When I asked Kwadwo if I could stay and learn from him, he answered with a twinkling smile, "Only if you marry me! The gift must remain in the family."

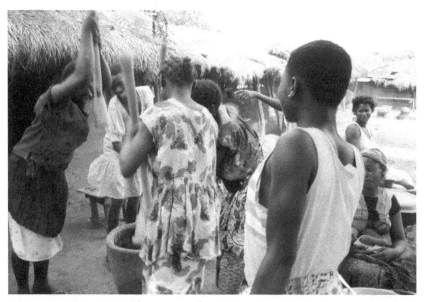

Women in Upper West, Ghana, pound corn in a mortar.

I said I was tempted, and Alec laughed to think of me uprooting my life to come here and live in a mud hut. I liked seeing how the strengths of tradition, customs, and skills had been handed down through generations, much more firmly rooted than Western medicine, which seemed poorly transplanted. For example, modern Western-trained midwives were taught to deliver women on their backs, unlike the traditional birth attendants who knew that village women preferred the safer squatting position. It wasn't surprising that women favoured delivery in their own homes and villages.

In Tumu, Alec met a boy named Joseph and was proud that he could speak with him in French to trade addresses. All the kids in the schoolyard came out to see Alec show them how to ride a bicycle, which was owned by the schoolteacher.

We stopped in a village called Hamile and crossed the border into Burkina Faso to shop for fabric for the project's nursing staff uniforms. Alec loved another chance to use his French. At night we slept in an unused hospital ward, carefully squatting in the adjacent field the next morning, since there were no water or toilet facilities in the hospital. It was still morning when we moved on to the village of Kokoligo.

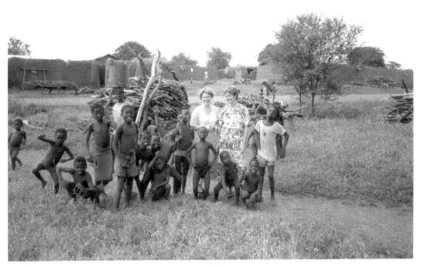

A meeting with villagers in Upper West, Ghana.

Normally, rural villagers worked their farms early in the morning, so community visits had to be made prior to 7:00 a.m., before people left for their *shambas*, which could be some distance from their homes. That day we were staying later because the community was in mourning for an elder who had died. His funeral took place around us as we drank beer and sat on log benches under a tree. After being taught by the village chief, Alec practised throwing the last few drops of *pitoh* onto the ground with a slapping sound. I wasn't sure if drinking low-alcohol beer from a calabash at eight in the morning with his mother constituted the kind of extra educational experience Alec's grade six teacher had in mind when she agreed to let him come with me for a month. But this was the funeral of an important village elder, and Alec was having the time of his life.

The recently deceased man was seated on a chair on a platform up near the trees. He was dressed in traditional clothing: a blue woven smock and trousers. The dead man carried a bow in his left hand to hunt for food on the way to the afterlife and a calabash in his lap for water. Women, I was told, only needed a calabash, which made me wonder if the food taboos in village life, where men got most of the protein, carried over to the afterworld. Alec glanced up at the deceased respectfully. This was the first dead body he had ever seen. And his second funeral. The first had been when he accompanied his father to Bear Island in Lake Temagami in northern Ontario when Doreen Potts, the wife of Chief Gary Potts, had died.

We, too, had our calabashes of *pitoh* and ate groundnuts. The smell of roasted meat and nuts, along with the scent of smoky fires, hung heavily in the morning air. It wasn't too hot yet; the air still felt fresh. We sampled tasty morsels of roasted chicken from huge platters of food that had been prepared and discreetly contributed money to help pay for the funeral expenses. Men and women, on opposite sides of the platform, danced in mourning to wooden xylophone music. Roosters pecked carefully for dropped crumbs of food. Dense green trees surrounded the village clearing.

The dancers and musicians, together with the men and women selling food and beer, wore red-and-black clothing in mourning. They were already a little tipsy from sampling *pitoh*. Still, their bare feet found the ground firmly as they kicked up dust.

After the funeral, we returned to Wa. Early the next morning Jens took us to Mole National Park, a game preserve. He explained, "Alec, this isn't a tourist attraction. It will be extremely hot, and there will be insects everywhere. There are no sheets, so we'll use torn curtains to cover us at night."

The next morning a light mist drifted in the high canopy of leaves formed by the tall trees. We were on foot. Jens wore khaki trousers, a brown belt, reddish-brown leather shoes, and a favourite powder-blue short-sleeved shirt. A Ghanaian guide led Alec, quietly and calmly, toward the animals. Jens and I stood a little behind them. A few feet away we spotted wild antelopes gracefully bounding through the trees. A family of seven elephants, three adults with four smaller young, moved heavily through the bush, reddish dust on their bodies from a cooling roll in the mud, occasionally snorting, then tossing their trunks upward to eat from leaves above their heads. Wild boars with curved tusks and bristly brown fur hurtled through the grasses off to the right. Alec spoke no words, but I could see the amazement on his face.

On the way back to Wa, Alec saw traditional healers selling medicines in French by the road. Again he was able to practise the language. His eyes grew wide as he read out the names of the diseases on the pictorial signboards.

When we prepared to leave Wa, Alec was sad. "I'll have to leave my friends, the cook, Abu, Abdulai, the man at the reception, the guard, and the cleaners. Now they understand I haven't been brought here for an arranged marriage with your friend Evelyn. I'm only eleven!"

Reluctantly, Alec got up at 5:00 a.m. for our departure and tearfully said goodbye to Abu. He watched cautiously as Dominic stopped on the way to Accra and bought live snails threaded on a rush string. When the time came, Alec could barely say farewell to Jens and his wife, Diana.

Later on the plane as we flew home, my son told me, "I'm glad I came. I like the way children live here, how I lived. I felt more like myself here. And, Mom, you're different here than you are at home. The stars here are also different than they are in Canada. I wonder when I can come back." Seeing Ghana through Alec's eyes changed how I saw my work.

In looking at "quantity" — deaths or health of children — I had been missing some important aspects of quality. I had been measuring diseases and the success of interventions to save children's lives. What might have mattered more was the joy of the children who greeted us as we came into their villages, laughing and dancing with great mischievous smiles. How could I measure the generosity of the poor street child who gave me a perfect rose in Bangladesh when I rushed busily past her?

Alec had bloomed in Ghana, thirstily drinking up the simple warmth of the people who had accepted him, not judged him on his school performance or his athletic ability. In our affluent Western culture we lacked some great gifts. The children in Ghana were well behaved, respectful, hard-working, and brimming with life. Just as my life had been brightened by the African women who gathered me into one of their dances or sang on the way to get water while heavily burdened, Africa had lit up Alec's spirit.

ETHIOPIA, 1994

The Jeep travelled along the dusty road, carrying our team of two Ethiopian and two Canadian physicians. We were thinking about the coffee ceremony the night before, the beans slowly roasting on a fire while we waited, tantalized, the smell of burning incense mixing with the aroma of pungent coffee. But today was about work. We were discussing how best to strengthen primary health care in order to reduce the death rates of rural poor children when we spotted the body of a small boy lying on the road. Men and women, many barefoot, went about the business of subsistence living, carting foodstuffs, water, firewood, and farming utensils. Carefully, they stepped around and over the child while flies gathered on his face. We were unsure whether he was dying or dead, for he made no motion to push the flies away.

I suggested to the driver that we stop. My Ethiopian colleagues and the Canadian who had three years of experience here told me that was foolhardy, and they related several stories of being stopped in similar circumstances, only to be beaten and stoned and barely able to escape. Was the boy a decoy, placed to entice us out of the car to be attacked and robbed? Was this happening because we were strangers? For some reason had this child been deliberately harmed and left there? Was there some type of retribution we didn't understand? Or was this like a big-city scene where people avoided assisting a victim out of fear of the costs of getting involved? I never found out, nor did my Ethiopian colleagues who, as affluent urban physicians, were in some ways as culturally isolated from this rural community as we Canadians were, separated from it as we were by income, tradition, and lack of hardship.

A few miles farther along the road a cow had fallen. Ill? Exhausted? Suffering from the heat? Other cows stood in a circle around their fallen friend, making shade with their own bodies so that even I felt comforted by their presence. White birds on the backs of the cattle, egrets hitching a ride, had joined the circle. It was such a contrast with the human scene we had passed earlier.

Ethiopia continued to have poor care for pregnant women and high death rates for children under five.[14] While Ghana had more political stability, Ethiopia had continuing civil war and frequent leadership changes, which undermined progress in basic health services. I was now training public health workers without Jens, on a project funded by the Canadian International Development Agency (CIDA).

When we arrived at our destination two hours north of Gondar, we were welcomed into a round sun-baked mud-and-stick home. The medical students were working with designated community members as part of their training concerning the problems of poor families. As part of our evaluation of the students, we interviewed the family. They told us how helpful they had found the students. One of our Ethiopian colleagues translated as I told the mother how well cared for her children were. I thanked her for her time, admired the small baby on her breast, and mentioned my own children. Once this was translated, she turned with tears in her eyes. Crying quietly, she spoke to my colleague in Amharic. The reference to my children, who were older, had reminded her of her two teenage children, whom she hadn't seen since they were airlifted to Israel ten years earlier.

Seeing my confusion, the mother and the translator told me how the Falasha ("stranger" or "exile" in Amharic) Jews in this northern region of Ethiopia were evacuated to "safety" in the promised land of Israel during the civil wars here. In 1984–85 (Operations Moses and Joshua), and again in 1991 (Operation Solomon), with the assistance of the U.S. government and the CIA, thousands of Ethiopian Jews were "repatriated" to Israel from camps in Sudan to which they had fled, and from Gondar, Ethiopia.[15] Families were separated, since people didn't understand what they were agreeing to when lists of Jews were drawn up. The Israelis modified special Hercules planes, removing the seats in order to crowd at least two hundred people per aircraft for the evacuation. This woman's husband and children went as part of her brother-in-law's extended family. She was left alone and hadn't seen or heard from them for the past ten years.

Subsistence society, however, was shaped around the family. Those who weren't selected for the evacuation re-formed family units. This woman's new husband, the father of the beautiful baby she was now suckling, had also lost his wife and children in the airlift. Now these two people had become a new family, mourning together the ones who had been taken away.

Teams of Israeli psychiatrists had come to Gondar to learn about Falasha culture and to understand the Ethiopian Jews in exile in Israel who hadn't fit easily into their new culture. No one, it seemed, had thought of trying to reunite families, and with the creation of new family units, such reunions would never take place.

We returned to Addis Ababa the following day. As part of our evaluation of this Canadian-funded project, the current director hosted a small party. One woman I met that evening, a Canadian psychologist, told me she was having trouble adapting child development tests to the Ethiopian context. How could a child bond to a cuddly doll, she asked, when the girl was frightened by the ones the psychologist used because dolls were unfamiliar objects? The psychologist was studying attachment between mothers and malnourished children to see if the mother rejected the child who was thin and had a lesser chance of survival. Starving families had to make difficult choices. Mothers might have to decide who could survive. Their work was made more complicated by national decisions that limited food availability. Land that could be cultivated for food was relegated to grow coffee or *khat*, the recreational drug widely used and sold to neighbouring countries for good profits.

Politics seeped deep into the soil in Ethiopia. Each new government dismantled the previous governments' ministries and agencies, often damaging the entire health system. Each new regime uprooted community volunteers who helped with immunization so that vaccination coverage fell drastically, taking years to return to previous levels.[16] Additional preventable deaths of children from diseases such as measles, tetanus, and tuberculosis added to the civilian casualties of war.

The civil war that had deposed Mengistu Haile Mariam in 1991 was over, and donor countries flocked into Ethiopia with aid projects. But donor assistance was also shaped by politics. A bureaucrat could decide to change the geographic focus of our aid, or drop the health sector, or end the association with an implementing partner.

Canada withdrew from the health sector in Ethiopia, contributing only humanitarian food aid. Canada's major project in the health sector saw a large share of the budget go to overseas fellowships for senior doctors. Those doctors were linked to the former Mengistu regime, and for personal and political reasons they didn't return to Ethiopia once the government changed. The goal of training public health doctors abroad was for those doctors to return and become teachers themselves to train others in a newly established school in Ethiopia. And the money for the fellowships would also benefit the Canadian sponsoring university. But in the end, Canada and Ethiopia lost out. American and British doctorates and master's degrees were seen as more desirable than Canadian ones, and jobs overseas were more attractive than anything in Ethiopia.[17]

The support that Canada gave to public health worker–training schools in Jimma, Gondar, and Addis Ababa was phased out once the project came to an end. However, support was provided by other development partners so that achievements could be sustained. Contributions from a range of donors pooling their support to the health sector ensured that after peaking in 1990 at 20 percent of children dying before the age of five, the rate of deaths of children steadily fell in Ethiopia.[18] This trend has continued. Still, while there has been a doubling of the numbers of women delivering with a skilled attendant, this is only now 10 percent, and three times more urban women than rural ones deliver safely. And just over half of Ethiopian children are fully immunized, again with large rural/urban disparities. It is difficult to fully assess immunization progress as estimates of coverage vary widely; for example three doses of diphtheria tetanus pertussis was cited as 37 percent, 63 percent, and 86 percent by different methods. The lower rates reflect the lack of skilled health personnel.[19] The need for improved maternal and neonatal health care continues in order to build on the gains of saving the lives of children between one month and five years of age.[20]

There are many hopeful initiatives in Ethiopia. For example, the Hamlin Fistula Hospital in Addis Ababa repairs women with obstetric fistulas (tearing from vagina to bladder or rectum) from unattended obstructed labour. Most of these women have stillbirths. This focus on care for poor marginalized women hasn't only addressed fistulas but has helped to prevent the problem by improving maternal and neonatal health services. The Hamlin Fistula Hospital has become a model of care, and several other countries, such as Nigeria, Sudan, Bangladesh, and Tanzania, have established similar facilities.[21]

Specific services in Ethiopia such as fistula care and prevention serve as successful examples, and the country also boasts of general improvement in health indicators. In the early 1990s, indicators of poverty, malnutrition, and basic health in Ethiopia were among the worst in the world, with widespread hunger and food insecurity, a literacy rate of just over one-quarter of the population, fewer than a third of children in school, and a high infant mortality rate (deaths of children under one year). The rates of infant and under-five mortality steadily improved and had fallen a further 25 percent since the Demographic and Health Survey of 2005. By 2016 the under-five mortality rates had fallen almost another 50 percent to 58.4 per 1,000 live births. Interventions to treat childhood illness such as oral rehydration show little difference by income quintile; 31.5 percent of the poorest receive oral rehydration compared to 37.3 percent of the richest. In contrast, 4.3 percent of the poorest quintile have secondary education compared to over 30 percent of the richest.[22,23]

Now Ethiopia is one of the target countries, based on its own government's commitment, to receive support from a special UN Maternal Health Thematic Fund that aims to improve coverage by midwives to reduce deaths of pregnant women and their newborn children.[24] Skilled birth attendance doubled between 2000 and 2011 from 5 percent to 10 percent and more than doubled to 26 percent in 2016.[25]

NIGERIA, 2015

In the Muskoka Evaluation of Canadian support to mother-and-child health, Nigeria was one of the focus countries and was noted to use a mix of strategies to save the lives of these vulnerable groups. In terms of child health, we looked at deaths of children under five, infants under one year, and newborns up to one month of age. In the decade between the Nigeria Demographic and Health Surveys of 2003 and 2013, deaths of children under five dropped more than 35 percent, from 201 to 128 deaths per 1,000 live births. By 2016 the under-five mortality had dropped even further, to 66 per thousand live births. Deaths of children under one also dropped by 50 percent from 2000 to 2016, from 97 to 48 deaths per 1,000 live births. But Nigeria is highly privatized — 65 percent of health-care providers are for-profit and in the private sector. This contributes to inequities in access to care. For example, although there is a policy for free artemisinin-based combination therapies (ACTs) for children under five and pregnant women, for treatment of malaria, since 2010, there have been widespread stock-outs of ACTs in Nigeria causing an equity gap with poor people using cheaper and less effective monotherapies.

The decline in neonatal deaths was a more modest drop of just over 20 percent, from 48 to 37 per 1,000 live births, reflecting the need to improve maternal health (Nigeria 2013 Demographic and Health Survey Key Findings).

Globally, over one-third of neonatal deaths or deaths in the first month of life took place on the first day of life. Nigeria accounts for 9 percent of the global burden of first day deaths.[26]

Fewer than 40 percent of Nigerian women have a skilled birth attendant or post-partum care, and there are wide urban/rural and socio-economic variations. Three-quarters of women cited at least one barrier to getting care. Half had no money for care. One-third could not travel the distance to health care, would have no transport, and feared there would be no health worker available or no drugs for treatment. One-fifth feared no female health worker would be there, or they could not get permission from their spouse, or they feared to go alone. Cultural and health systems factors are clearly closely integrated in the medical challenges of saving children's lives.[27]

4

I HAVE NO EDUCATION:

CHINA, BOTSWANA, UGANDA, AFGHANISTAN, AND NIGERIA

CHINA, 1996

An eight-year-old girl was wearing the most improbable outfit: an embroidered hot pink velvet dress and white satin blouse, which would have looked at home on a Ukrainian folk dancer. But she was dressed in the traditional clothing of the Yi people, one of China's minorities. She sang a song of harvesting; behind her the cloud-filled sky reached down to touch a mist-covered mountain. A party of twenty or so Yi people dressed in lavish headdresses and similarly brightly coloured and embroidered tribal outfits had come to meet us at the border. Our team of two, Yuwa Wong, a health economist, and myself, were the first foreigners ever allowed into this part of Yangbi County, Yunnan Province, in southwest China. We had made our way in a long procession headed by a police car with flashing lights. The Yi offered small glasses of alcohol to toast the occasion, with ceremonial handshaking by the governor.

Yuwa and I were here to assess the health needs and resources of this area in order to plan a mother-and-child health project to be funded by Canada. Having left Canada during an onslaught of media hype about the treatment of Chinese orphaned girls, I had expected the worst — girls left to starve in orphanages and high rates of selective abortion of female fetuses after women confirmed the gender of their unborn children through ultrasound. Yet at every step of our journey the hospitality was generous, the openness and spirit of trust genuine. We had been sung to, presented with gifts, and welcomed, with more warmth as well as more organizational efficiency than I had experienced in any of the other twenty-four countries I had worked in by that time. That isn't to say there weren't problems in China. But considering the odds, China was on its way to achieving a miracle.

The overall health status in China compares favourably with middle-income countries, and education is a high priority for families and government. China has worked hard to achieve universal education. The rate of illiteracy among youth and young adults has been kept below 4 percent, over 90 percent of the population has achieved the universal nine years of compulsory education, and government contributes heavily to support education. Progress is evident even in remote and rural parts of the country such as Yunnan Province. In these poor areas, families send their children to school for at least nine years.[1] Minority peoples living in rural areas are allowed three children.[2] Adults have high levels of both literacy and numeracy.

Poorer health exists primarily in underdeveloped and remote regions, which is what brought us to Yangbi County in 1996. In spite of strong gains in female literacy, the county had higher death rates for women and children than elsewhere in China, which induced the Chinese government's request for Canadian support.[3]

We were invited to a celebration one night. The constellation Orion, my familiar travelling companion, was overhead. Sparks flew into the dark sky from huge bonfires in a central courtyard. The air in this mountainous region was cool, fresh, and lightly lemon-scented. Small children played around the fire and threw short sticks into the flames, reminding me of the Indigenous communities in Canada where I had worked. The kids played in the same free, wild-spirited way.

There were speeches of welcome and then a round dance where dancers moved in a circle with carefully orchestrated steps — again similar to Indigenous communities. The men and women sang to one another, the men with deep voices, the women's voices clear and very high. Young, unmarried people engaged in this courting song — the first step toward planning to marry was to be sure they liked each other's singing.

Two women in tribal dress beckoned me forward with their own welcoming faces, asking me to join the dance. With a slightly nervous smile I got up from my seat on a log near the fire. The dance was simple, but it was still difficult to do. I found it hard to follow the steps. Faces flickered in the firelight, and the onlookers clapped their hands with encouragement as my feet felt the rhythm — left foot overlapping in front of the right as we kept sidestepping to the right, then changing to move in the other direction. Yuwa laughed from his safely seated position.

I was smiling broadly now, unable to speak in any shared language except for the dancing. My two partners grinned as I followed their steps more easily. It seemed there was no time but this moment; I never wanted to leave. The dance drew slowly to a close, and I was led, laughing, back to my seat by the fire.

It was the turn of other team members to sing. I made a short speech, introducing our translator and another colleague from the Provincial Health Bureau. They sang a Chinese love song in beautiful, unrehearsed counterpoint harmony. The head of the County Health Bureau, to express his happiness at our visit, sang "I love my Dali," about his hometown, paraphrased from a song from the Peking Opera. The head of the Epidemic Prevention Centre sang a modern love song. Everyone appeared to know the words and sang along with him.

Then it was time to return to traditional dancing. Half of the group assembled to dance around the fire, while the singers moved to the other side of the courtyard where karaoke had started up. An ancient dance form competed with the video screen and loudspeaker.

This mix of old and new, traditional and modern, industrialized and undeveloped, is part of the complexity in China where there is a very high standard of living and exceptionally modern health-care facilities in some areas. Health risks associated with births in very young or older women, or with births spaced too closely together, have been eliminated by the acceptance of family planning and later marriages and pregnancies (see Appendix 3). The family-size policy is one, two, three: one child in urban areas, two in the rural areas, and three allowed for ethnic minorities. Perhaps because of the matriarchal nature in some of the ethnic cultures we were visiting, there didn't seem to be any gender discrimination (such as neglect of female children). Yet in other parts of the country female children still filled orphanages, abandoned so families could try for a son for their one child. By 2015 the one child policy was relaxed to allow two children, due to gender imbalances from abortions of females and an ageing population.[4]

Poor rural areas such as Yunnan weren't able to compete with the economic bustle affecting much of industrialized China. In the past, rural villages provided for their health workers who performed basic health care for free. Now these communities had little money. In these poorer regions, health services were minimal. Babies were delivered at home in unsanitary conditions, and they suffered high rates of easily preventable or treatable conditions such as pneumonia and diarrhea.

The following day we visited a township hospital staffed and patronized by tribal minorities. They wore their traditional dress topped with bright turbans in different colours: some black, some floral orange, some floral pink. The blouses were white, with red vests over them, and white belts. On the vest a complex chevron of diagonal stripes (two different blues, one pink, and one orange) moved from left shoulder to waist. Blue trousers or skirts completed the outfit.

The Provincial Maternal and Child Health (MCH) adviser had close-cropped black hair and a white lab coat and was studiously professional. But she had tears in her eyes as she showed us her patients on the ward. Zhang Li had given birth alone at home. Hemorrhaging, she then walked five miles to reach the hospital. Post-partum hemorrhage was the leading cause of death in this area, affecting the poorest women who had delivered at home without medical assistance. Zhang Li was convinced to stay in the hospital with an hour of urgent reassurance by the mother-and-child health doctor that the town would pay for her stay.

An excellent doctor from the same national minority told us about her experiences delivering babies and promoting health education and prenatal care in remote villages for those women unable to get to the hospital. "But even when they get here, you see how poor we are at the hospital? You see that the patients are sleeping two to a bed? Last year we had no beds until our own hospital director made them himself out of wood he had cut from the forest."

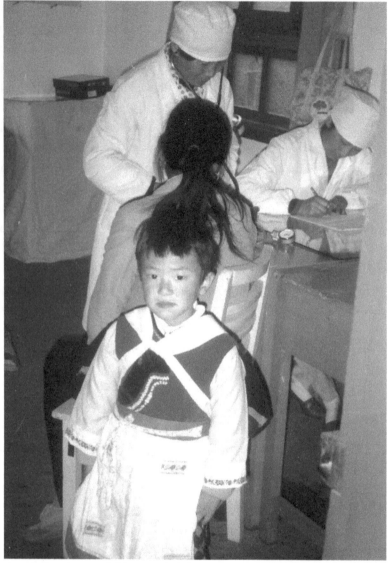

An ethnic minority child in a tribal clinic in Yunnan Province, China.

The next day we travelled to a village clinic staffed by a "barefoot" doctor who specialized in traditional Chinese medicine. He had a wide array of herbs and roots that he had collected himself. His clinic was busy. He worked with another doctor who handled the maternal-and-child health.

She introduced us to an admission she had made that day, a woman with extremely high blood pressure and swollen ankles who was being treated for pre-eclampsia. She had been driven to the hospital by tractor. The village doctor had paid the hospital fee.

We were a large group. We had five people from the health directorate of Yunnan Province, four doctors from the county, three from the township, our own translator, Marianne, who could translate our English to Mandarin or Cantonese but needed an additional translator for the local dialect, and Yuwa and me. Someone from one of the departments was videotaping our procession. Carefully, we picked our way up a mountain path. The view was expansive: terraced rice fields with small village houses nestled within them, smoke curling lazily in the cold mountain air. We visited three families in a village at the top of the hill in their courtyard as roosters pecked in the dust and one fat pig strolled sleepily by.

Small bare benches were brought out, and Yuwa and I were welcomed as "coming from the land of Norman Bethune thousands of kilometres away."[5] This became a refrain repeated time and again to introduce us.

We learned that women used to deliver babies alone at home on the bare ground but now went to the village doctor. This was a huge transition; in so many other poor countries, women could only afford to deliver at home with an untrained birth attendant. The average per capita annual income in the region was under fifty dollars. The people were poor, with insufficient food to eat, but all of the children were in school. Families slept in two rooms on bare wooden beds without even a blanket against the cold. As I had seen in Nepal, the homes were often shared with animals if the family was rich enough to own a pig. Animals in the room or under a house were a great source of warmth when it was cold.

The hospitality we experienced was simple and generous. I felt my soul respond at the most basic personal level, beyond the buffers of material protection and status that characterize our many human interactions.

We knew it would be at least a year or two before any Canadian project found its way to bring resources to this area. So Yuwa and I tried to give a personal donation to the township hospital to help honour their commitment and enable them to continue to subsidize care for the poor. The people refused. They explained that the fact we had come from "the land of Norman Bethune thousands of kilometres away" was enough, and they were already ashamed they had no gifts for us. And yet the villagers around the hospital had been up since dawn picking wild mushrooms from the forest so that we could be welcomed with a wonderful meal. Only by invoking the memory of Bethune, who was generous with his time and resources, were we able to get them to accept our money.

Later that night, back at the county seat, ballroom dancing replaced karaoke and dancing around the bonfire. Apparently, this was a legacy from Mao Zedong's time, where a tradition developed of weekly ballroom dancing for party brass. Our team, plus local officials, health workers, and hotel staff, joined in. Although this was an area foreigners had never visited, the bizarre mutations of cultural contact were still present. I felt as though I had gone halfway around the world only to arrive in Cobalt, a small northern Ontario town near my own where karaoke and open mike nights are popular in the local bars and where ballroom and line dancing are taught in the local arena one night a week.

The next day, the flashing lights of a police car once again led our procession of cars back to the county border. Unlike other poor countries where I had worked, where cries of "*Baksheesh!*" from countless beggars entreated you for charity, the poor in this region seemed untouched by contact with affluent nations. They had yet to be corrupted by tourism. How soon before this would be a place where all transactions — social, economic, political — must be accompanied by bribes?

At the border the Yi people greeted us anew. They sang, toasted us with wine, and presented us with farewell gifts. One official handed us woven bags, beaded hats, and slippers.

We drove for hours through mountains and small villages, with an orange and an apple on the dashboard of the car. Our driver had placed them there for luck. The winding roads could be treacherous, with the possibility of both landslides and numerous careless drivers. The Chinese character for apple is similar to the word for safety, and the character for orange is like the word for good fortune, so the fruit were there to ensure our safe travels.

At each stage of the journey throughout Yunnan Province, health workers gave us impressive factual presentations of the situation of maternal and child health, complete with English translations in carefully summarized printed reports that showed how meticulously they had kept statistics on children immunized, births and deaths, numbers of children treated for illness, mothers attended in pregnancy. I had never seen this level of educational sophistication in remote health centres in other developing countries.

We noted more women in leadership roles such as county governors, and more leaders among ethnic minorities in each region than I had seen in any country, including Canada. In each region the majority of health workers were from the ethnic minorities of the area. Seventy percent of the traditional Chinese medicine doctors in one hospital were women, as were 95 percent of the medical and nursing staff in the county hospital.

In other countries, such as the former Soviet Union, the increase in the proportion of women in the medical profession has reduced the status and earnings of doctors. The same has been seen in China. But there has been an additional change in China, as well as more women coming into medicine: the inroads of a capitalist ethos to health care. There has also been a shift from a communal system, where health workers gave freely of their skills for a share of farming produce, to one where their skills are sold in a privatized system that gives little value to public health (immunization, antenatal care) and high value to services such as medically unnecessary intravenous infusions of vitamins and antibiotics.

As we travelled, the stunning landscape added to the intensity — the great flowing Yangtze River, the Jade Dragon Mountains, the Black Dragon Lake. We saw so many different styles and colours of housing and clothing as we visited each indigenous minority. We saw eight-hundred-year-old towns with great carved doors and ancient stonework brimming with history but untouched by tourists.

One night we heard a traditional ethnic concert of Nakhi music. The leader of the band, imprisoned for twenty years during the Cultural Revolution, claimed to be sixty-seven but looked about forty. He said music was medicine for the soul and made you young. Five members of this group were over eighty. Four young Nakhi women had recently joined the band. This was a radical change for a music form preserved for centuries by Taoist monks dating from the Tang Dynasty and historically monopolized by men. It was so exciting to feel these shifts — educated women now in positions of authority in politics and health care, and making inroads in culture. Such a paradox! With the one-child policy, many female babies are aborted, and yet there are such strong roles for the women who are lucky enough to be born.

But after the magical time in Yunnan, and in its beautiful cities such as Lijiang, it was disappointing to come to Beijing, where we had to negotiate the project with national officials and with the Canadian Embassy. Beijing was in the midst of threatening preparations to acquire Hong Kong and was sabre rattling in the straits off Taiwan. Here I could feel the presence of the senior party officials who had allegedly embezzled vast sums of money. What of those hard-working, well-educated friends in the poor rural provinces?

After six weeks, I returned to Canada. I thought about the Indigenous Peoples' experience in Canada and the disparities we, too, have within our own country, with news blackouts on the appalling living conditions of First Nations. We, too, have had charges of bribes and corruption against former prime ministers. Perhaps things aren't so different here. In the poor rural Canadian North, we, too, live on the margins, like the ethnic minorities in Yunnan Province. We, too, have higher death rates. Our tribal minorities also have worse health conditions and lower educational achievements than the dominant white culture.[6] As they have in China, Indigenous Peoples in Canada are starting to assume greater positions of leadership. So I thought it was fitting that Canada had chosen to support a mother-and-child health project in a part of China that faced some of the same challenges as my own country. We could learn from each other, and the project would ultimately contribute to reductions in deaths of children and pregnant women.[7]

But one huge achievement in China is education. Literacy rates in China are high for indigenous people. And there isn't the huge gap between male and female literacy rates seen in most poor countries. So many factors work together for maternal health. High female literacy reduces deaths of pregnant women and children under five. Educated women are more able to access family planning, which is universally promoted in China. Educated women have more power to gain an income. In many countries, including those in the developed world, the poor are dominated by female-headed households where poor women with little education and poor employment try to raise children.

Still, women are an underclass, evidenced by the decision of families to abort their female children when the government allows only one child. This social challenge will require more generations to change, and the educated women of China can help to work for this transformation. Nevertheless, when women in so many countries aren't able to be educated past primary school, where the national priority is slow to subsidize education for girls, it is remarkable to see a country that has recognized the importance to the economy, and to health, of female education.

BOTSWANA, 1998

China has succeeded well in educating its population, including its minority peoples. Still the country's indigenous people have lower incomes and higher death rates for pregnant women and children. China has a GDP per capita income of just under $8,000. Botswana's GDP per capita income is almost double that at just under $14,000, (it had risen further to $16, 220 by 2012) but the same disparity is seen with the ethnic minority peoples in that country.[8] Botswana also has a high national priority for literacy, with a rate of more than 80 percent,[9] yet the San people or Bushmen are only 25 to 30 percent literate.[10] The pattern of inequality in Botswana has persisted but is improving: the level of inequality is the world's third highest.[11]

Botswana is a wealthy country, rich with diamond mining. Instead of the fourteen dollars per person spent every year on health in countries such as Tanzania or Uganda,[12] Botswana, with a population just under two million, spends nearly one thousand dollars on each man, woman, and child.[13] And there are serious health problems: 22 to 23 percent of the adult population is HIV positive.[14]

This level of funding has provided for many interventions such as midwives at birth, family planning, and emergency obstetric care to reduce the deaths of pregnant women. Over 95 percent of women deliver safely. Botswana is one of only three countries in Sub-Saharan Africa that has been successful in family planning. The number of births has been reduced by more than one child per woman in just over a decade. Almost half of the population uses contraception.[15]

In 1998, after my assignment in China, I was in Botswana as part of a UNICEF project. My task was to work with the schools, health services, and NGOs to develop an adolescent sexual and reproductive health strategy for the country. While the literacy rate in Botswana was high, many girls were leaving school as teenagers, since it was compulsory for a girl to quit school if she became pregnant. The fathers of their children could continue at school with no penalty. It was very difficult for teenagers to get access to contraception, even condoms, which would have helped prevent HIV. UNICEF was attempting to find ways to allow girls to prevent pregnancy and HIV and to stay in school if they did become pregnant. We also had to target our strategy to specifically meet the needs of ethnic minority groups such as the San people.

Travelling by Jeep to Francistown, I was amazed. This was a new Africa for me. Roads were paved. Very few people wore traditional dress, and Western suits and dresses dominated. The shops were filled with luxury goods and spare parts, and there were a few Zimbabweans with money who had crossed the border to search for supplies unavailable in their own desperately struggling nation.

But mining had also brought HIV in addition to wealth. Despite Botswana's outstanding achievements in maternal health and education, it has the second highest rate of HIV infection in the world, after Swaziland and Lesotho.[16] The close links to diamond, gold, copper, and nickel mines, and the sex workers that surround the mines, had increased infections of local women. In Francistown, a city with a population of 93,000, 55 percent of pregnant women were HIV positive.[17] Nationally, one-third of the sexually active population was estimated to be HIV positive, and the life expectancy had fallen to forty years because of AIDS.[18] Half of Botswana had premarital sex, but only one-tenth had access to condoms. And for kids under twenty-one, it was against the law at that time to get tested for HIV.[19]

In a well-equipped school in Francistown, I asked the principal about the possibility of youth-friendly, school-based clinics where adolescents could access contraceptives and learn about HIV prevention. After all, the majority of infections occurred in young people. He glowered and firmly rejected this idea. "This would just encourage them to be promiscuous," he said. Then he added, "Of course, we have to expel a girl if she becomes pregnant. We can't tolerate this immorality in the school."

At the YWCA I found a more encouraging response. They were trying to establish peer counselling where adolescents could teach one another about reproductive health. Mosalagae Tlhako was angry and gestured wildly with his long fingers. "Sixty percent of the population in Botswana is under thirty years of age. Nearly half of the people living in this country live in female-headed households. The high proportion of HIV cases occur in people in their twenties, so infection started when they were teenagers. Teen pregnancies and sexually transmitted infections in adolescents are rising. Many young girls trade sex with their older married boyfriends to pay their school fees. We have to involve the schools!"

As part of this assignment, I was looking at diverse groups of adolescents. In-school and out-of-school youth had different needs, and we would have to develop various ways to reach them. Kids in school could be supported with clinics at or near their places of education. Unemployed youth could be helped through recreational facilities. If adolescents had jobs, there could be ways to reach them through their work. The San would need a strategy supportive of their culture.

Like China, Botswana is a multi-ethnic country. Like China, the literacy rates are high.

But some groups such as the San have far lower rates of literacy and higher rates of pregnancy and death in children and pregnant women than the Tswana, the majority ethnic people. So working with the San required specific attention.

I left urban Francistown and headed off to the west and south across the Kalahari Desert, which comprises nearly three-quarters of Botswana. *Kgalagadi*, from which the name Kalahari is derived, is a Tswana word meaning "the great thirst." Like in Ghana and Sudan, we seemed to travel in our four-wheel-drive Jeep for countless hours and see no one. Only the occasional circular pans of shining salt, from several hundred metres to several hundred kilometres in diameter, broke up the great expanse of arid and sandy ochre-coloured soil. This was home to the San who comprise 1 percent of Botswana's population.

In 1998, the year of my UNICEF assignment, the majority (twenty-five hundred) of the San was removed from their ancestral homelands in the Kalahari. It took four years before the process was completed in 2002 when all access to health, water, and education was removed by the government of Botswana from the ancestral homelands of the San, forcing them to relocate outside the Kalahari reserve.[20]

UNICEF tried to ensure some culturally sensitive programming in the midst of this compulsory eviction. Dr. Stephen Simon, then the resident representative for UNICEF, explained, "Our primary aims were to improve the abject conditions of the student hostels by developing a new model structure that could be readily converted into classrooms in the future should the hostels no longer be needed. We also established twinning relationships between some Basarwa [San] schools and elite ones in [the country's largest city] Gaborone."

This, however, required San children to board over sixty kilometres from their families or walk nearly ten kilometres to school. It reminded me of the Indigenous students in Canada and Aboriginal students in Australia who were forced to stay with white families in towns far from their own communities in order to receive a Western white education. San children struggled with Setswana and English, the languages taught in school.

Dr. Simon clarified, "We endeavoured to introduce San language instruction with Setswana in the lower grades and created a mentoring system pairing older and younger students. We tried to make the teaching curriculum reflect more of the world in which the children lived; re-engineered the academic year to accommodate the participation of the children in their families' traditional hunting and gathering forays; and involved the parents to a much greater degree in their children's schooling. We also offered a study tour for Ministry of Education officials to Australia so that they might learn about more enlightened approaches to 'Aboriginal' education and tried to plug Basarwa kids into emerging international Internet networks of indigenous children."

The government claimed it was removing the San so it could improve their living conditions, including enhanced access to education and health services. Officials consistently denied that access to potential diamonds was a factor (there is one mine on the edge of the Kalahari) and instead argued there was a compelling need to establish a game preserve on which no traditional hunting could be allowed. The Oppenheimer family of the DeBeers mining group, partners with the government of Botswana in the Debswana diamond mining interests, owns the large Tswalu private game reserve in the Kalahari. The San were settled in camps and were provided, ironically, with limited access to water and basic services such as health and education.

The education system in Botswana is centrally controlled and not tolerant of the cultural diversity of groups such as the San, who have an informal traditional system of education and respect for elders. In 1995 only 18 percent of school-age San were in any form of education.[21]

Teachers often have different cultural backgrounds from their students, and the corporal punishment common in schools is forbidden in San culture. So without culturally sensitive possibilities for schooling, the San remain further behind, with higher death rates of mothers and children and greater poverty.

Madala, a San student, and his sisters wore khaki drapes, which didn't cover their breasts. They sported coloured beads around their necks and wrists. When they spoke with one another in their home, they used the clicking sound common to Khoisan languages. They turned to me to explain how cut off they felt from their traditional lives as nomadic hunters. "We are one of the oldest cultures on earth! We have lived here for over seventy thousand years."

Their brother cast a more intimate light on their problems. "We are called Basarwa, a Tswana word meaning 'not quite human, inanimate, original dwellers, or people without cattle.' It was legal to kill us until 1948. We are looked down upon. How can we compete in school? If we are taken away from our culture, we will become drunk. We have high rates of unemployment. We will not respect our women and will start to have casual sex. These habits are not in our culture.

"Our traditions are the most ancient in the world. We have learned to live sustainably in a difficult environment. We are losing all of this. The world is losing all of this, in order that we go to school. We need to find a way to support unique cultures such as our own while we gain an education."

UGANDA, 2002

Minority cultures globally face challenges in health and education. Few countries have been able to meet the specific educational needs of unique cultures. Health customs are also culturally bound — giving birth, raising and helping sick children, educating the young, and gender roles are highly linked to traditions that have evolved over generations.

The Ugandan medical superintendent led us into a grass hut, one of nearly fifty built closely together around the *kraal* (an outer wall of thorny bushes and an inner wooden wall), which protected the livestock. A little sorghum and a spinach-like vegetable grew outside the hut. One old grandfather, Moses, sat by the smoky fire, with grizzled greying hair and a brief plaid wrap around his waist.

"*Ejoka!*" we greeted him ("Hello" in Ngakarimojong). Through our excellent translator, whose Christian name was Mary, he spoke. "I fought for the British in the Second World War, against the Italians in Ethiopia. The British knew we were good fighters. But the government of Uganda wants to take our arms away. Unlike Sudan. Sudan gives arms to our brothers the Toposa. They know this helps them with the fighting in southern Sudan. The rebels, the Sudan People's Liberation Army [SPLA], have also given arms to the Toposa. They both know it is good to have the strong skills of our people of Turkana on their side. But you, woman, why are you here? Why are you with this *amusugut* [white woman]? Why are you not with your family?"

He had addressed this question to Mary, the translator. Although when I met her in Kampala she wore Western clothing, here she was in traditional dress. She was tall and slender, with heavy earrings, a great array of yellow beads around her neck and, a blue-and-white-and-burgundy-striped open wraparound coat over her red plaid dress. She turned to me. "It's hard for me to be here. My family didn't want me to go to school. I had other duties — to help with the family, to collect water from a spring several kilometres away from our home, to grow food in our garden. I had to fight to get where I am today. Let's leave this man."

But he wasn't finished with us. "You, woman, you have dishonoured your family. Do you have children? A husband?"

Mary turned again to me in the dark, smoky room, which was starting to make our eyes a little teary. "When I was at school, only one-third of girls my age became educated; only one in five went on to high school.[22] Most of my friends were married off when they started to menstruate. There are so many soldiers now. They have sex with the young girls. It lowers the bride price."

Moses was angry that we were speaking English with each other and that Mary wasn't answering his questions. But they still seemed to see some things the same way, though they had made different decisions about how to overcome the problem. Moses shouted, gesturing wildly. "You went to school! We must not let our girls go to school. The teachers and the boys have sex with them, and then we cannot get good bride prices for them. We must keep them in the community where we can protect them."

Mary, who now had a master's degree in sociology, was one of the young people who attended secondary school between 1988 and 2000, a time when there was a great increase in the numbers of young people in secondary education. But this region, the Karamoja, wasn't sampled. The districts were too unstable and prone to violence for statistical teams to visit, and the rates were so low they brought down national averages. The Uganda Bureau of Statistics had been limited in its ability to tailor surveys in the Karamoja. While the region is more stable politically, it is the most food-insecure area in Uganda: 45 percent of children under five have chronic malnutrition and 7 percent have acute malnutrition.

The Karamoja is an arid savannah region in northeastern Uganda bordering Sudan, populated by semi-nomadic cattle herders. I was travelling with Mary and Robert, the medical superintendent, over heavily rutted roads along grassy grey-green plains dotted with occasional thorn trees to visit Karamojong villages. Our two battered Jeeps lurched down the road accompanied by police escorts (UPDF — Uganda People's Defence Force) because of the political instability. No other vehicles were visible. A gentle, cooling breeze tempered the hot, dry air but carried a fine brown dust that settled in our clothing. Fine fluffy white and grey clouds weighed heavily against an azure sky, and soft ochre hills flanked the front of Mount Moroto in the distance.

We were here to learn from the villagers themselves: how they gave birth, how they planned their families, what their worries were about their health and their families. Our goal was to develop a special package of reproductive health services that would be shaped around the specific culture of the Karamojong. Several districts — Kotido, Moroto, and Nakapiripirit — were going to receive additional help from Denmark (Danida) because these communities had higher rates of maternal and child deaths, as well as lower literacy rates, especially for girls, than elsewhere in Uganda. Complex formulae based on these factors showed this region to have the highest human poverty index and the lowest human development index in Uganda.[23]

The medical superintendent explained, "The Karamoja is still recovering from a famine in 1980 that wiped out a fifth of the population and more than half of the infants under one, but now the population is growing, family planning is seldom used, and the influence of Christian churches is strong. The Karamojong are cattle raiders. Life is based on cattle for which women are traded. Guns [AK-47s] to help steal the cattle are needed. Raiding guns and cattle elevate a man's status and help him to secure women. Cattle raiding is also a rite of passage for a young man. This ethnic group originated in Ethiopia hundreds of years ago and is linked with the Maasai in Kenya and Tanzania, the Toposa in Sudan, and the Turkana in Kenya."

After my detailed project development work, Danida decided against such a support, that giving money in a block to the whole health sector would be sufficient. But since then in the Karamoja, HIV rates have more than quadrupled from 1 percent to 5.6 percent, while nationally rates have decreased to under 8 percent.[24] The low literacy rates and low status of women are seen as factors in high deaths in pregnant women and the HIV rise. HIV campaigns can't use posters since few people can read, and condoms aren't available. One component of the rejected project was to create a system of community-based distribution of contraceptives. According to United Nations Population Fund, Deputy Representative Dr. Hassan Mohtashami, 1 percent of women in the Karamoja use contraception compared to 18 percent nationally.

There has been a reduction in adolescent pregnancy[25] in the country as a whole, with a drop from just over 40 percent of teenage girls who had started having children in 1995 compared to only 25 percent in 2006.[26] The rate is relatively constant. In 2016, 25 percent of adolescent girls have begun childbearing according to the Uganda Demographic and Health Survey 2016. But this hasn't occurred in the Karamoja, which translates, as it does throughout the globe, to higher maternal deaths as adolescent pregnancies are riskier. In the Karamoja the majority of females have had female genital cutting, and the majority were sexually abused in primary or secondary school by a male teacher. Girls with secondary education have their first child two years later than their uneducated sisters.[27] According to the 2016–2017 household survey, female literacy has increased: 30 percent of both males and females cannot read. But in the Karamoja, 65 percent of women can't read.[28]

And women with no education have nearly eight children each, their educated sisters just over four. Every new pregnancy brings with it the risk of death to the mother, and births spaced too closely together bring death to newborns who are born too small if their mothers are still breastfeeding the baby born before them. High fertility translates into higher rates of deaths of pregnant women. But women need education to understand these dynamics.

In 2009, the deputy representative for UNICEF, Dr. Gloria Kodzwa, told me, "One problem that faces adolescent girls in schools is a barrier so simple we seldom think of it. Adolescent girls start to menstruate and have to use a clumsy system of rags. They are teased and become embarrassed. It is easier to hide this 'shame' by staying home and carrying on domestic tasks for the family instead. So they fall behind and drop out. UNICEF has been providing sanitary kits for these girls." We went on to discuss the problems facing girls in the north of the country where rape was common, where many women had been captured as sex slaves by Joseph Kony and the Lord's Resistance Army. Sixty thousand children have been abducted in northern Uganda in the past two decades — many taken to Sudan where the boys are trained as soldiers and the girls as sex slaves. Dr. Kodzwa, clearly fatigued by problems that have seen so little progress in northern Uganda over the decades, explained that more than

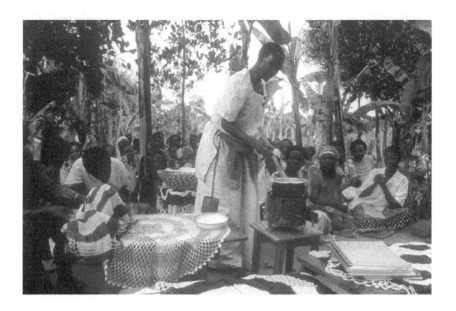

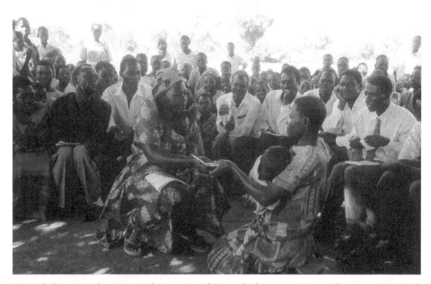

Female literacy classes in other parts of Uganda have encouraged women to teach one another, not only numeracy and literacy, but also basic health education, such as how to cook more nutritious food, so they can better care for their children when they are ill. This is an example that can still be utilized better in the Karamoja. In some cases, medical assistant students come from their schools in Mbale or Fort Portal, Uganda, to learn from the villagers.

40 percent of the schools in war-torn Kitgum district were closed; many students were simply studying under trees, and 85 percent of the schools that were open were in desperate need of repairs and school supplies. While the 2006 ceasefire has made the region more stable, rebuilding will take time and resources. Innovative solutions are needed to educate over a million and a half internally displaced people in northern Uganda.

The region still has a net enrollment of 35 percent, far below the national average of 90 percent. But many improvements have occurred. The Norwegian and Irish governments have supported primary education using adapted models of education to support nomadic life[29] and the building of primary schools in the region.

The Karamoja remains at a disadvantage in Uganda today, with lower levels of education and higher rates of deaths of children and pregnant women. The same is true of the San in Botswana and the ethnic minorities of China. Carefully tailored solutions are required to improve education and health while supporting cultural and ethnic diversity. Respect for culture is crucial when we look at improving maternal health, since the roles of girls and birthing customs are so deeply embedded in tradition. When we try to impose national solutions or push for "improvement" such as forcing young minority people away from their communities in order to educate them, we break down fragile bonds.

Cultures in chaos have higher death rates. The broken communities of indigenous peoples in Australia and North America have high rates of substance abuse, adolescent pregnancy, violence, and death. In poor countries, small ethnic groups have even greater challenges, since there are even greater pressures to use the lands they inhabit, or to push the agenda of a ruling national ethnic group. If we are truly committed to improving the health and education situation of these most marginalized peoples, we need to work with great care and caution to ensure that we build on cultural strengths, rather than destroying them. And when we study national education rates, we need to scrutinize more closely the differences between groups that are blurred by aggregate statistics. The poor, including ethnic minorities, have lower rates of education and higher death rates for pregnant women and children under five.

Afghanistan and Nigeria, 2015

Since the end of Taliban rule and the installation of the transitional government of the Islamic Republic of Afghanistan in 2002, there has been a major investment in the education of women and the training of skilled female health workers. This increase in the number of trained female health-care providers has had a major impact on mother-and-child health. Between 2002 and 2012 there has been a threefold increase in the percentage of deliveries by a skilled birth attendant and a doubling of completed immunization for infants, but still half the women deliver at home and only half the children under two are fully immunized, with pockets of insecurity in the country making health care inaccessible. Polio is not yet fully eradicated.

By 2013, 28 percent of health workers in the public sector were female, compared to in 2002, when only 21 percent of nurses and 24 percent of doctors in the country were female. There are now more than four thousand midwives trained in the country and more than twenty-five hundred are actively deployed in public facilities, a more than tenfold increase since 2002. Canada's Muskoka support to Afghanistan included a strong gender strategy within its health projects.[30]

Education of girls is fundamental to improving the health of women and children. Cultural transformation to encourage communities to allow their daughters to be educated can be slow and difficult. Courageous women such as Malala Yousafzai,[31] who advocated for female literacy in her own country of Pakistan when her home was under the control of the Taliban and was shot and injured by the Taliban, are examples of this positive force for change. She survived, and some of the funds from the first edition of this book were directed to her non-governmental organization. But with change comes resistance.

In Nigeria, extremist terrorist groups have kidnapped girls attending school, held them captive, leading to the deaths of some and releasing others with threats to their families to keep them out of school if they want them to be safe.[32] This is in Borno State, where female literacy is the lowest. Nigeria was one of the countries which received support from the Canadian government in the Muskoka Initiative for mother, newborn, and child health. I had really wanted to go to Nigeria. It is one of the most high needs countries in the world. Nigeria accounts for the largest number of global maternal, neonatal, and child deaths (as the country contains one-fifth of the population in Sub-Saharan Africa). But the attacks by Boko Haram in the north were deemed too dangerous to allow me to travel, so this part of the evaluation had to be done as a desk review. So, if too dangerous for me, who else was being affected by the insecurity, kidnappings, and killings in the north?

More than 80 percent of women in Nigeria's southeast and southwest have skilled attendants at delivery compared to 12 percent in the northwest and 20 percent in the northeast. It is harder to deliver health care in the north. The numbers of girls getting an education are lower and family planning use is lower, which pushes higher the risks of teenaged pregnancy. Female literacy is an important determinant of maternal and child health: nearly half of girls aged 15–19 with no education have begun childbearing compared with 2 percent of girls with secondary education or more. Nine times more women with secondary education have a skilled attendant at delivery compared to just over 10 percent of women with no education. Education levels, as well as urban/rural differentials, affect the total fertility rate: rural women have an average of 6.2 children and urban women 4.2.[33]

According to the Countdown to 2030 collaboration, Nigeria faces the greatest inequities in access to reproductive, maternal, newborn, child, and adolescent health of all countries being assessed.[34] In our evaluation, in 2015, of the Canadian support to the Muskoka Initiative using 2014 data, there were wide discordances in access and utilization of these health services. Income inequality in a country, as measured by an indicator called the GINI coefficient, is a major determinant of deaths in children under five. (This is a method of assessing income distribution in a country, named for an Italian statistician Corrado Gini in 1912.) Illiteracy both causes and is a result of income inequality. As women have higher rates of illiteracy, a major strategy to promote female literacy would help reduce deaths of children under five. Literate women are also more likely to use family planning and skilled birth attendants, so this would also improve maternal health as discussed above.

Education of women is closely correlated with income, which again links to the use of reproductive health care. In Nigeria, as indicated by UNICEF's Multiple Indicator Cluster Survey 2011,[35] access to and utilization of basic health services across the continuum of care were compared across income quintiles, looking at the top and bottom 20 percent. Pre-pregnancy, rich women are twice as likely as poor women to have their demand for family planning satisfied. Four times as many rich women than poor women have four prenatal visits and are more than eight times more likely to have a skilled birth attendant at delivery. Rates of early initiation of breastfeeding and use of insecticide-treated bed nets are closer by income quintile, but coverage is still only approximately one-quarter of infants and children. Infants from wealthy families are four times more likely to be immunized against measles, diphtheria, polio, tetanus, and pertussis than poor infants. Vitamin A distribution and oral rehydration for diarrhea (which can be done by primary health-care providers, including immunization teams) also show wide discordance across income quintiles, but care seeking for pneumonia is three times more common for rich children due to the cost of health centres and medicines.

Overall there has still been progress. There have been achievements in family planning and child mortality reduction. Approximately every five years there is a national survey, the Nigeria Demographic and Health Survey (NDHS). The total fertility rate averaged across all income groups dropped from 6.0 births per woman, as estimated in the 1990 NDHS, to 5.7 births in 2003 and 5.5 births in 2013. Birth spacing is the most cost-effective intervention to save the lives of children and mothers. Gender disparities persist. Less than 15 percent of women in a union use contraception to delay pregnancy, only 2 percent more than in 2003. Twenty percent of women want no more children compared with 12 percent of men, with men wanting on average two more children than women want. Women are less able than men to make family planning decisions. In the 2016–17 Nigeria Multiple Indicator Cluster Survey, just over half of pregnant women have been immunized against neonatal tetanus, less than one quarter of children 12–23 months have been fully immunized, and 60 percent of women compared to 70 percent of males can read a short sentence.[36]

Investing in female literacy is an important strategy that is sustainable and helps promote cultural change and improve the demand side of reproductive, maternal, newborn, and child health.

TANZANIA, 2018

After initially deciding to ban pregnant girls from attending school, during and after a pregnancy, the government of Tanzania agreed to work on a plan with the World Bank in late November 2018 to allow pregnant girls to continue their education. The World Bank had stopped a $300 million education project to Tanzania upon learning of the initial Tanzanian government decision to ban pregnant girls from an education. In mid-November 2018, when the World Bank initially withdrew their aid, Denmark, the second largest donor to Tanzania, followed. It withdrew $10 million in foreign aid after the Tanzanian government enacted the ban on pregnant girls' education as well as a homophobic crackdown in the country. Denmark may divert another $6 million to NGOs.[37]

5

WHY ARE WOMEN DYING GIVING LIFE?

INDONESIA, ZIMBABWE, BHUTAN, BANGLADESH, ZAMBIA, TANZANIA, AND PAPUA NEW GUINEA

INDONESIA, 1998–1999

Outside, the clothesline was strung between palm trees that leaned beside the stilted home. A goat, two chickens, and a sad looking dog lay sleepily in the shade below the stilts. Squares of cloth — orange, brown, white, beige wraps to cover lower bodies — shook gently as they dried in the breeze. The roofs in this fishing village were heavy thatch, cone-shaped. The walls of the homes were upright wooden boards shaped to surround circular huts. The ground between the homes was stony and strewn with shrubs. Barefoot kids laughed on the path between the houses. Large rush-woven baskets, wider than the length of my arm, waited for grain. Women in headscarves sat chatting with each other in the next compound, holding their babies and occupying themselves with the simple rituals of preparing food for their families. Bright red flowers bloomed at the very top of a brilliant green tree.

At the water's edge below the village, fishermen prepared to bring in the day's catch, the men moving surely with nets and poles, and pushing the long, narrow vessels out to catch the waves. One man, who seemed quite old, with wiry legs and lines on his face, stayed behind to mend a torn net. Another older man repaired the thatched roof of a hut four buildings away. On the shore I saw three other village women, two, it seemed, with babies in their arms as the wind rushed past them, blowing those long, loose skirts while they leaned and gazed out to sea to where their men worked to bring fish to the table. They were clothed in long colourful dresses with long, flowing white headscarves.

I ducked my head to enter the home. I was with Merpati, a *dukun bayi*, or traditional birth attendant. She had delivered the newest member of the family, a boy named Wayan (First Son), one week earlier and had brought me to this Sulawesi village in Indonesia to see the naming ceremony of this newborn. The home was carefully swept and tidied, with a few treasured belongings stored neatly.

"*Ibu!*" the family called out, welcoming the traditional birth attendant as they would a mother or some other honoured member of the family. We had brought coconut milk to wash the baby's hair for the occasion. Our contributions to the ceremonial feast were brought out of our bright crocheted bag with care: chicken and spicy peanut sauce for satays, bright red chilies that we had selected at the market earlier in the morning, a small selection of fish and melt-in-your-mouth velvet tofu. A bowl of water with a slice of lime was set before us to wash our hands before eating. The family had roasted a goat to share with the guests who were joining them in welcoming the new son.

The *dukun* was missing a tooth on the bottom right side of her mouth. I could just see the space. Her eyes crinkled as she smiled and explained with gestures and a few words how she had given herbal drinks to Nirmala, the new mother, said prayers with her, and massaged her abdomen to ease the labour pains. When the baby arrived ten hours after the start of labour, Merpati had cut the cord with a bamboo knife and had put turmeric on the umbilical stump to help it heal. With her help, the *adik-adik*, or placenta, had been buried away from the house, since the child had been a boy.

Merpati had stayed with the family to help with household chores, to ease the burden on the new mother. For a poor family in Indonesia, the *dukun* is affordable. To help with the delivery she would be paid five thousand rupiah (about one American dollar when the Indonesian economy collapsed in 1998) and a bag of sugar or uncooked rice. In contrast, the cost for a midwifery-assisted home birth was an impossible four times more money, and ten times more for a normal hospital delivery. Emergency obstetric care, such as a Caesarean section, could cost a year's family income.

Nirmala still seemed tired. Shyly, she beckoned to the *dukun* to talk privately in Bahasa Indonesia (the 250 languages of Indonesia have now blended into a common one that also has traces of Arabic). She lifted her saffron head scarf and whispered to Merpati. Nirmala was still bleeding heavily and was worried. Merpati took Nirmala to the back of the room and placed her on a bed. I stood in front to shield them a little while Merpati examined the new mother, and the guests moved quietly outside to the courtyard to give them more privacy.

Merpati was also worried. Nirmala was soaking the rags, which had been collected for her lochia, the bleeding after birth, but the amounts were much greater than usual. Merpati felt the womb; it wasn't contracted tightly as it should have been. Nirmala was concerned that Pontianak was near, a spirit woman who had died in childbirth from bleeding. It would be important to get help soon; at night evil spirits could harm them if they travelled.

The nearest *puskesmas pembantu*, or health sub-clinic, was two hours away. A smaller *posyandu*, or health post, was only an hour off, but some of the necessary drugs might not be available. We had visited it yesterday and had seen that stocks were low. There had been locally produced intravenous fluids, antibiotics, and some oxytocin for bleeding. Small, slightly grubby packets of Indonesian-made contraceptive pills and injections of birth control that can be given every three months for nursing mothers, had been lying on the shelf. And in the supply cupboard were even more birth control pills, which had a constant turnover because there was a high demand for them. Women now only had three kids each instead of six. Cheerful posters flapped on the wall of the *posyandu* — *DUA SUKUP* ("two is enough"). This had been a popular slogan since Suharto's time, in the late 1960s. The message wasn't only to help Indonesia deal with the pressures of over two hundred million people living on six thousand islands but was also an effort to save the lives of pregnant women. One percent of the women who get pregnant in Indonesia will die — two every hour.[1] The easiest and least expensive way to save these women's lives is family planning to safely space births at least three years apart.

Merpati knew the family relied on her; she knew there was a problem, but she also knew she didn't have the skills to do anything. Had some of the afterbirth been left behind when the baby was born? Usually, hemorrhaging after a birth takes place in the first two days, but it can occur later.

Could Merpati ask Wulandari for help? She was a *bidan di desa*, a village or community midwife, one of more than fifty thousand who had been trained in the previous ten years in Indonesia to help reduce the deaths of pregnant women. And if Wulandari helped, would the family still pay Merpati her five thousand rupiah? Could the family afford Wulandari's assistance?[2]

Merpati beckoned to a nephew, who looked about ten, to find Wulandari and ask for help. She would stay with Nirmala, caressing her brow, murmuring prayers. I checked Nirmala's pulse, which was rapid but regular and still strong. Merpati explained to the family, to Nirmala's mother and husband, that extra help was needed because of the heavy bleeding. The naming ceremony would have to be postponed. Money might be needed for the midwife.

Wulandari arrived within twenty minutes with medicine — oxytocin.[3] She greeted the family and asked Nirmala to put the baby on her breast to help tighten the womb to slow the bleeding. When breast milk is released, so is a hormone that contracts the uterus. Wulandari rolled Nirmala onto her side to inject her in the buttock. Then she asked the family to get Nirmala ready to travel to the nearest health sub-centre. The family was a bit uncertain to be receiving so much help but thanked Wulandari. "Terima kasih banyak," they said shyly.

"Kimbali. Tidak apa apa," replied Wulandari, brushing aside their thanks with a gracious "You're welcome. It's nothing."

Three hours later Nirmala was in a bed with an intravenous line running, and the bleeding had stopped. A small piece of the placenta that had been left in the womb had been carefully removed with gloved hands at the clinic. Nirmala could have easily died.

I was working for the Asian Development Bank, helping several provinces on the island of Sulawesi to outline what they needed to do to reduce the deaths of pregnant women. Between trips to the provinces I had to travel to Jakarta, Indonesia's capital, to meet with other donors such as the World Bank to ensure all of our projects were coordinated. Outside my window I heard army soldiers marching. Riots had limited where we could travel. Daily bulletins from the embassies advised the safest routes. The politicians we met as we tried to negotiate support and funding from the development banks to help strengthen health care for pregnant women in rural villages were known for the percentage they took from every contract.

After debating the issues of support, I left for Lampung, a province in Sumatra, to help design strengthening of primary health care. Indonesia has wide inequalities in basic health services, since some islands are far wealthier than others. This was an attempt to allow individual provinces to bring money to their own level, bypassing Jakarta.

I spent the early evenings gazing over terracotta rooftops and at the sea, islands, and hills in the distance. I could have been in the Mediterranean with palm trees beneath violet skies. I reflected on the peaceful, well-ordered rhythms of Indonesian villages carried out in homes of grass and leaves, bamboo and mangrove poles, and the currents of life linking families with the land and sea. I thought of Nirmala, who could have lost her life except for the help of the *bidan di desa*, who had been trained through the support of other countries. I was grateful I could help bring this kind of aid. At night I saw hundreds of dancing lights — oil lamps on bamboo buoys calling forth the fish to come sliding through the water and into the nets.

What currents pulled me? Was I the fish or the lamp? How did I learn to listen to the calling voices of Nirmala and her sisters? Did I follow and lead at the same time?

Wide gaps between rich and poor in Indonesia mean many areas have worse health care for pregnant women and their children. Jakarta has death rates about one-quarter of those of poorer provinces, yet Jakarta controls the flow of money for health services to the different provinces. Poor supplies of equipment and drugs in some areas, untrained traditional midwives who face problem deliveries on their own, a failure to realize when a pregnancy or delivery is becoming a high risk, and problems transporting emergency cases to centres with adequate support all compound the problem.

Family planning has been quite successful in Indonesia, and the country makes the most of the contraceptives needed in the country. This is the cheapest way to save women's lives. Still, poor women can't afford midwives to deliver their babies safely, and the untrained attendant they can afford lacks skills as well as connections to the health system to mobilize emergency obstetric care. So the pilot project that Indonesia initiated to train the *bidan di desa*, a community-based but skilled birth attendant, was a huge breakthrough. In fact, it has become a model that other countries, such as Bangladesh, have followed. Although the deaths of pregnant women had been falling in Indonesia, the midwives left rural areas for more lucrative private practices — 50 percent of maternal deaths take place in only five of Indonesia's thirty-three provinces[4] and the country is still not on track to meet its targets to reduce the deaths of pregnant women.[5]

ZIMBABWE, 1999

In 1999 Jens Hasfeldt was diagnosed with prostate cancer and began treatment. He asked me to replace him on a mission to Zimbabwe, a country lurching toward disaster with a teetering economy, worsening death rates of pregnant women and children under five, and HIV rocketing out of control. I would be working with a Belgian, Leo Deville. I caught him smiling over our first breakfast while I was in a midstream torrent of ideas. "Okay," I asked somewhat sheepishly, "what did Jens tell you about me?"

"That you never stop talking!"

Leo was also a public health doctor, and we were trying to plan a large financial support program from different European governments for Zimbabwe. This involved a lot of risk, since many of the European governments lacked confidence in their Zimbabwean counterparts, and there was always the possibility of corruption in the handling of such a large pot of money. One way to reduce the risk would be to channel a large percentage of the cash to NGOs and faith-based facilities.

Faith-based hospitals provide services for the poorest and most vulnerable in most developing countries, often supplying approximately half of the national hospital care. As part of this project, Leo and I were to visit various mission facilities to make sure those facilities continued to receive funding from such government-to-government programs.

Our first stop was a cash-strapped mission hospital, which was welcoming an important visitor. Father Michael was sleek in his finely cut suit, amusing us with tales of his business-class flight from the United Kingdom to Johannesburg and a stopover at the Victoria Falls Hotel. "Wonderful! The setting! The food! So beautifully refurbished! And only US$230 a night!" We were discussing whether his employers — an affluent order of nuns — would buy, as a tax deduction, this debt-ridden hospital.

The hospital's aging chief of staff, a German surgeon who had come to Africa after the Second World War, had struggled to keep things going, encouraging volunteer doctors to come and help, trying to scrounge drugs and supplies, often working as the only surgeon on call day and night for Caesarean sections and other acute cases. But she was worried: there were few young doctors coming to Africa to dedicate their lives to the mission hospitals, and it was hard to get operating funds from the government to run faith-based facilities. The poor she was trying to serve in this rural area didn't have the money to pay for hospital care — for normal childbirth assisted by midwives in health facilities, for emergency obstetric care when women during labour or delivery developed complications, or for costly diseases like AIDS.

The Zimbabwe government was now charging for previously free maternal health services, and the missions were receiving smaller grants from the government for their facilities. The death rates of pregnant women in Zimbabwe had doubled in the previous ten years, according to independent assessments,[6] which was partially related to the HIV epidemic but was also a result of the shortages of midwives and doctors and impossible fees. So the chief of staff had jumped at the chance to discuss the hospital's needs with this visiting priest, a "godsend," she was sure.

Father Michael seemed excited as the chief of staff told him about the grave financial difficulties of the hospital. "Actually," he said, "it's everything we need. You say it keeps losing money?"

Well, yes. The three of us explained about the ongoing economic crisis in Zimbabwe, the cost of hospital care that forced pregnant women to die at home or arrive at the hospital with no money and leave the mission further in debt, the heavy toll of AIDS and tuberculosis.[7] This was, after all, a Catholic mission hospital.

It was hard to believe our elegant visiting friend was a priest. He was so vastly different from our short host, Father Brendan, who worked in the parish that had the hospital as its centre. Father Brendan, an enthusiastic football coach with a thick Irish accent and a heart of gold, usually wore rough sandals and an old burgundy T-shirt over his small paunch. He had been in Africa for years as a brother and had decided to study for the priesthood in Ireland so he could return as a priest to serve the poor.

Leo Deville and I had only been working in Zimbabwe for two weeks. With every passing day we had become more depressed at the corruption and incompetence. We agonized over the collapse of the country, the hardships suffered by the former middle class, and the lack of basic care for pregnant women and the sick and dying. "Land reform" was a land grab that had simply reduced the amount of food being grown, causing people to go hungry. No dissent was tolerated. While we were safe as outsiders who weren't politically involved, Zimbabweans weren't free to give any opinions about the government. But many priests like Father Brendan were actively helping the poor.

Our delegation of "development partners" had met Father Brendan in our first week in Zimbabwe at a health conference, where his knowledgeable questions and utter frankness had impressed us. He had stood up at one of the meetings to challenge the government when its officials had stated they wouldn't provide an inexpensive drug called nevirapine (an anti-retroviral drug against HIV/AIDS) to pregnant women to prevent newborns from becoming HIV-infected by their mothers during birth. The government had argued that its policy wasn't to create more AIDS orphans. "So it's better to let both mother and baby die?" Father Brendan had shouted incredulously.

Father Brendan understood health problems better than the district medical officers. He could quote the statistics and give reasoned priorities for the scarce health funds. He could explain responsibly the need for better trained workers. "We simply don't have enough midwives! Why should they stay here when their salaries aren't paid?"

Better than anyone he knew the sleazy politics at the top — the crooked deals, the money embezzled by politicians, the people who feared for their lives if they opposed President Robert Mugabe. But he also recognized the strong possibilities for change at a community level with the right support and leadership. Working as a parish priest, he had visited all the health facilities in his charge from small grassroots clinics to the referral hospital and had volunteered in each one. Leo and I were both only occasionally practising Catholics. Father Brendan's dedication almost brought back our own faith — faith in humanity, faith in God.

When he spoke passionately about the importance of distributing condoms to adolescent girls — "poor wee things, they have no rights whatsoever" — I had asked, astounded, if he was really a priest. A Catholic priest? "Surely to God, girl, you don't think we should just be letting them all die of AIDS? And if you ever saw a thirteen-year-old girl die from a septic abortion, you'd know I'm right about this. You're a public health doctor. You must know that contraception saves the lives of pregnant women and children under five by spacing births."

I decided that now wasn't the time to mutter that it wasn't me he needed to convince but the leaders of our own church.

Father Brendan had also mentioned, in passing, that the bishop was beginning to wonder about the annual rate of marriages in his parish. "Why do you have more annulments than marriages?" Father Brendan had been asked.

"Well, you know, once the women tell me about the beatings — I won't stand for that in my parish! The husband either changes his ways or he's out! That's it! So I just annul the marriage. As for the unmarried women, the older men are just after the young girls and then the girls fall pregnant, and the men won't leave their wives. So they either end up pregnant and alone, or they die trying to kill the baby. Or they get infected with HIV by their boyfriends. Some men even believe that sex with a young virgin will cure their AIDS. No, I ask too many questions and not many are able to stand up with the right answers."

Leo and I accompanied Father Brendan on his visits to Catholic clinics in his diocese (all well stocked with condoms). I asked the staff at one if they distributed condoms to unmarried people. They glanced at Father Brendan before answering, just in case we were senior emissaries from one of the mission benefactors.

"Oh, to be sure, you can tell them the truth," Father Brendan said, pointing at one of the cartons of condoms he had brought to the clinic for their already crowded storeroom.

"Father, where am I to put these condoms?" the Irish sister in charge asked him.

"Oh, Sister, 'tis true you know nothing. 'Tis the man who puts on the condoms, not the woman."

As we travelled, Father Brendan told us about the huge lands given by Mugabe to his cronies, the safari lodges for the rich owned by the even richer, all of which provided no revenue to the cash-strapped regions we were in because the president had exempted the lodges from paying tax. We saw the appalling lack of quality in the local clinics where most of the staff hadn't been paid for months. Mugabe was using the public treasury to pay the army to protect his share of the blood diamonds of the Congo, which was beset by civil war.[8] His personal greed was putting the operating funds for government social programs at risk.

The mission clinics that managed to beg, borrow, and steal were a little better off. Father Brendan had humiliated private mining hospitals into giving up all kinds of resources. He had twisted arms and refused the sacraments. Once, in the midst of a malaria epidemic, Father Brendan even threatened to bring all the dead bodies that were rapidly accumulating to the mine owner's palatial house if he didn't free up the mine hospital morgue for them. Father Brendan chuckled as he recalled these ruses.

He had so many skills in so many different areas, from carpentry to health care, and was so well read and reflective that he was truly a Renaissance man. Father Brendan told us how he, himself, had delivered babies by tying the cord with a rosary string and how he had once given a ride to a woman whose baby was brought into the world in the back of his pickup truck at night by a blind old grandmother who had needed no light for her task.

Entranced by his stories, we rode for miles late at night when we knew we shouldn't be travelling, over roads unencumbered by cars, the stillness only disturbed by gazelles, chattering monkeys, and slow-moving elephants.

———————◆———————

Our journey with Father Brendan had brought us to this lunch at the mission hospital, discussing tax breaks with Father Michael. Our prospective benefactors, Father Michael's wealthy order of nuns, had built hospitals on land in Ireland that had proven highly profitable once sold. And even their operating hospitals were making money. "We have excellent quality of care, and people will pay for quality. In fact, we think we'll bring medical teams down here for a week or so."

We were curious. "Medical teams? What sort?"

The visiting priest replied that he thought plastic surgeons would be good. They had great ones in their Dublin hospital. He described how fun it would be for the visiting doctors to stay in the Victoria Falls Hotel en route. Father Michael, himself, would love to come back and accompany them. He represented the order of nuns, after all. They would own the mission hospital. He would be a valued member of the team. His eyes lit up as he described the falls again.

We asked, "Do you have general surgeons or obstetricians? TB or HIV specialists? Midwives?"

Father Michael didn't think so. He shook his head, no doubt wondering why we were asking, his brow wrinkled in thought. We tried to remind him about the kinds of health problems normally seen here. We had taken him on a tour of the wards, the overcrowded beds full of the dying, the women delivering on the floor. No, he didn't think they had tropical medicine specialists, either.

Leo and I, and the German surgeon, caught one another's eyes with questioning looks. Even cherubic Father Brendan, who had been so sure this was the fairy godfather who would wipe away all the debts of the hospital so it could go on serving the poor, seemed puzzled. Could this really be possible? Father Michael served no God the rest of us knew or understood.

"Well, actually, we don't really want to lose money, which we would if we paid those debts," Father Michael explained in his carefully modulated accent. "It's a tax write-off, you see. It just looks like it loses us money." He had grown up in South Africa and gone as a priest to teach theology in Dublin. Slick, flashy, proud, and self-absorbed, he was such a contrast to Father Brendan, who had made the opposite migration from Ireland to Africa.

Outside it was hot, with just a little breeze. Birds floated lazily on gentle air currents. A kingfisher glinted against the sun as it swooped toward the water that we could just see through the restaurant windows. Its back was blue, its underbelly bright. After the Flood, the kingfisher, sent by Noah seeking land, flew too close to the sun. Its breast was scorched red, but its back took on the hues of the sky.

I felt overloaded with the cumulative despair of fighting so many losing battles. In Zimbabwe, not only did the mission hospital we had visited not receive funding, but the large program support to the whole health sector that Leo and I had planned was also cancelled when the European donors, the development partners, lost all confidence in Zimbabwe. Smaller, more focused projects took its place. The work we had done felt largely wasted.

Sometimes, despite bad governments, donors can make a difference. In Zimbabwe it has continued to be a terrible challenge to help effectively. Much of the money that comes in is wasted, little gets to the bottom, there is worsening poverty, the health system is in a state of collapse, and death rates of pregnant women increase. In 1999, deaths of pregnant women had increased 140 percent over the previous five years.[9] Some areas such as rural Mashonaland had less than 45 percent of women delivering with skilled help, about half of the rate in the capital of Harare. Home deliveries with an untrained birth attendant increased nationally from less than one-quarter in 1998 to just under 40 percent in 2009 — women simply couldn't afford to deliver with a midwife.[10] The worsening poverty and deteriorating health system, compounded by HIV, has contributed to these shocking increases.

But there is some momentum in family planning for both educated and non-educated women. Without this the situation would be much worse. This progress continued. From 2010 to 2015 the average number of births per woman dropped from 4.1 to 4.0 and the use of modern methods increased from 57 percent to 66 percent. After peaking in 1999, the levels of infant and under-five mortality have dropped back to their levels from the 1980s. Sixty-five percent of pregnant women in 2011 had four prenatal visits and a facility birth; this has increased in 2015 to 75 percent for each indicator. And there have been continued supports to reduce HIV, which has led to great improvements: in 1999, HIV prevalence was 26 percent — in 2017 13.3 percent of adults were infected with HIV.[11]

BHUTAN, 2000

The number of deaths of pregnant women was nearly halved in Bhutan, unlike in Zimbabwe, where it had more than doubled in the preceding ten years.[12]

How could a country achieve this? Even if over half of the deaths of pregnant women still occurred at home, how had Bhutan increased the percentage of women who received the care of a "skilled birth attendant" from 15 to 23 percent and increased the use of contraception from 18 to 30 percent in just ten years?[13] How much of this achievement was related to the fact that literacy for women had doubled from 15 percent to over 30 percent, from 1980 to our visit in 2000, and how much to the improved availability of health workers to deliver babies safely? If Bhutan could do this, could other countries? Bhutan had received the Sasakawa Health Prize in 1997 (founded in 1985 to acknowledge outstanding achievements in primary health care) for a pilot project on primary health care in Mongar Dzongkhag, and had developed an impressive network of health facilities throughout the country. I desperately needed to see a success story in a challenging context.

Tshering, the auxiliary nurse-midwife, brought me down the narrow corridor to a small room off to the right, which had a slightly slanted ceiling.

A woman named Pema lay on the bed with a baby wrapped in soft green blankets cuddled to her breast. Tshering smiled, and Pema's face shone.

"I delivered her last night," Tshering said. "I am so proud. This is the one hundredth baby I have brought into this world. I have only been trained since two years. I went to the Royal Institute of Health Sciences in Thimpu. I am so happy to be working for my king, my country, my people. I am honoured that I am using my education, my gifts. When I was young, I had a long barefoot walk to school. It was Father Mackey who first taught me.[14] There were no schools for my parents. Look what I have learned to do. This mother had started to bleed at home. Her sister was helping to deliver her. They carried her, walking for five hours to our BHU [basic health unit]. I was able to remove the retained membranes and give her oxytocin. I started that intravenous you see in her arm. She is alive, and I was privileged to help her."

Pema smiled sleepily. One hand stroked the black hair of her newborn daughter, while the other caressed her prayer beads.

As part of our journey, we were asked to attend the ceremony to inaugurate a new basic health unit. We drove past Bhutanese villages where houses were decorated with giant male genitals for joy. Red chilies dried on rooftops everywhere. To open this new clinic we had a hard, rugged drive on a rutted road. Denmark had built the health unit, its bright white walls enlivened with floral designs, its windows and doors framed by elegantly carved wood. At the end of our journey, we spent hours feasting with the monks and health workers on yak-butter tea, marijuana-fed pork, spicy cheese, and grain alcohol served warm.

The next day I was part of the ceremony. I sat praying with the community as incense-burning ceremonial smoke wafted lazily upward. Monks wound their way around in a circle to bless this new place. I walked slowly behind them, their incense lamps swinging in front of us as we made our way down the mountain to the clinic. I danced and threw rice as a blessing, the dancing to sanctify the future work of the clinics. The monks, with their musical instruments and blowing incense winding their way clockwise around the clinic, blessed its future work. The sigh of grace and supplication responded around us.

Kismet or fate had finally brought me to this misty Buddhist kingdom perched in the Himalayas. I was in Bhutan because someone else had broken her leg. Danida had selected Bhutan, along with Zimbabwe, as one of its priority countries for development assistance. So when one of their doctors, who had been working on a five-year health plan for Bhutan, slipped and fell and had to go back to Denmark for surgery, she needed to be replaced. My appointed lot was to carry on her work.

For years I had hoped and prayed to travel to Bhutan. I had first learned of the country after listening, riveted, to Dorji, fifteen years earlier at the Liverpool School of Tropical Medicine where we had been both students and lecturers. Dorji and another Dorji (a common Bhutanese name) were two of the first people to leave this closed mountain kingdom to go abroad for post-graduate programs to learn skills to bring back to Bhutan.

And now I was here in Thimphu, Bhutan's capital. After the corkscrew landing, on Druk air, into Paro's airport, I was still reeling from altitude sickness, which made me feel as if I were continuing to spin around and around. Everything echoed. I couldn't quite trust what I was hearing in natural conversation and felt drugged. Mindfully awake, I walked to meet Dorji, who was now the principal of the Royal Institute of Health Sciences, a health worker training school. We glanced at each other shyly when we greeted, asked after each other's migraine headaches, and shook our heads in disbelief to think of meeting fifteen years earlier in Liverpool. It was an honour to meet his family, who proudly showed me his graduation certificate from the Liverpool School of Tropical Medicine.

Walking to work seemed to help re-establish my equilibrium. I passed a monastery where I heard the chanting, chanting, chanting — rhythms so ancient. I took long, wandering routes and relished the sound of running water rushing around me. I saw everywhere the flashing turbulence of rivers alongside the paths, felt pulsing life caught in the water, and saw the prayer wheels spinning with the current while faded white, blue, green, yellow, and red prayer flags flapped and flipped loudly on the slopes of the mountain. My heart fluttered with the prayer flags, each step a meditation. I passed men and women with lined faces, their prayer beads turning and flowing through their hands. I followed the Buddhist precept and strolled clockwise around the temples, sending the prayer wheels fastened outside spinning with my hand as I passed. Seeing the burgundy-clothed monks, small boys, and older men, reminded me that for this community, lives were dedicated at birth to the flow of the spiritual forces in our lives. On some deep level, I felt instantly at home in this kingdom of just over half a million people, perched high in the Himalayas between India and Tibet, with Sikkim and Nepal to the west, and disputed territory between India and China to the east.

Slowly, over several weeks, I worked with my team of Bhutanese counterparts to define what they hoped to achieve in five years. I was working in a country with little visible corruption, where senior health officials cheerfully walked for days to visit health facilities and communities, where the king spent weeks touring villages and listening to his loyal subjects, then returned to tell the donor government that more money was needed for water and sanitation, saying, "This is the people's priority." When Danida withdrew funding in 1998 from India following that country's nuclear test, the donor made it available to Bhutan to finance this important need.

That same year, the same wise king asked for more money from "development partners" for Nepal, to help stabilize the region. Nepal was and is a twisted issue. The United Nations High Commission for Refugees holds over one hundred thousand people of Nepali descent, who claim to be Bhutanese refugees, in camps across the border in Nepal (some of these refugees have been accepted into Canada). Bhutan claims they were offered Bhutanese citizenship, which was refused, and they have therefore been repatriated to Nepal, their country of origin. Some of them have families still in Bhutan. Although their relatives have remained loyal to the king, they are slowly losing their jobs with no explanation, they never get promotions, or they are deemed ineligible for the national positions in multilateral (United Nations) or bilateral (donor governments) offices.

Even in a land boasting of development achievement with an official indicator for "gross national happiness," tribal loyalty simmers below and just above the surface. It is a delicate balance that the Royal Government of Bhutan must strike with its strong neighbour India, with whom it shares equivalent currencies and army manoeuvres, yet Bhutan is politically and spiritually linked to Nepal. Bhutan must also maintain political stability with China, even though Bhutan is spiritually connected with Tibetan Buddhism.

With its ten indigenous social groups and three main linguistic groups, Bhutan has had a complex history. In the west and central interior, the people are descended from Tibetans who moved to Bhutan in the seventh century. In the south live the people of Nepali origin (Ngalops), who arrived at the end of the nineteenth century. The three main languages are Dzongkha, spoken in the west and being promoted as the national language, increasingly becoming a mark of nobility and status and promising access to high-ranking civil service jobs; Sharchop, the oral Tibeto/Burmese language spoken in the east; and Tongsa, spoken in central Bhutan. Bumthang is also spoken in central Bhutan, home of the original royalty, and Nepali is widespread as the lingua franca. These difficulties of language influence the production of health promotion materials for mother-and-child health. Which ones are chosen for translation? Who will be left out if English, or Nepali, or Dzongkha are selected?

In between work sessions to assess the skills of health workers, watching classes in the training school, and observing the quality of care in the clinics, I visited monasteries, sitting cross-legged with the monks in their small rooms in buildings perched on the mountain face, the monks' bedroom interiors papered with pictures of Bollywood film stars. One of the monks was dedicated to UNICEF and worked full-time on water and sanitation and improvement of child health. He laughed when he told me about a visit from two of my fellow Canadians. The monk had travelled abroad and had seen Toronto. He described his visitors: "These guys were very Toronto. Urban chic! They were fashion savvy and muscle-bound." He camped up his voice as he imitated their manner of speaking. "They visited me and one of my monastic brothers, Kim Sherpa, who had just emerged from years of solitude and meditation. They were so glad they could give us some direction. They read our tarot cards and told us what to do next in our lives. Can you imagine? We were too polite to refuse them."

The way back to my room at Hotel Druk, in Thimphu, included long walks in the hills and visits to villages to drink *ara*, a hot alcohol drink that was wonderful on a snowy day.

Travelling throughout the country to visit health facilities, I saw that different parts of the country represented quite diverse challenges. There was still some unrest in the rich agricultural land in the south of Bhutan, from which the Bhutanese of Nepali origin had been repatriated to Nepal by the Bhutanese government. Schools and clinics were burned down. I required travel visas and had to follow a carefully designed itinerary to take me only to areas in the south that were considered stable. I had to have government permission for each leg of the journey, even though we were led by Bhutanese counterparts. Security was tight. I found one hospital near a hydroelectric power station still being constructed and tried not to look at the list of names of Indian labourers who had died creating power to sell back to India. On my visit to the wards, there were several Indian patients with paralyzed legs awaiting stabilization before being pensioned off with little money back to India.

Like Nepal, Bhutan shares the same immense challenges that are due to the great distances between its sparsely populated settlements and its health-care centres or schools. We had travelled for a full day to the east and were now at a basic health unit (BHU), where Tshering, the auxiliary nurse-midwife, and her two male colleagues (a basic health worker and a health assistant) provided primary health care. This was one of over a hundred and sixty basic health units in the country. All three health workers would walk for hours to do home visits without complaining. All could deliver a baby. All received their salaries on time. Although our visit was unannounced and we had arrived at the end of a long day, the staff members were still busy seeing patients.

We were greeted with polite, warm welcomes and tea. Proudly, we were shown the medicines and contraceptives that were available. A book, *Buddhist Perspective in Family Planning*, endorsed by His Holiness the Je Khenpo, lay on a small wooden table beside a conch shell. A photo of Her Majesty Queen Ashi Sangay Choden Wangchuck smiled at us, informing us she was the goodwill ambassador for the United Nations Population Fund.

She was one of four queens: four sisters all married to the king. I had met the queens during my first week in Thimphu. They had led sixty Bhutanese and expatriates on a walk down the mountain to raise money for a nunnery, while the teenage crown prince, wearing his *goh* (traditional clothing for men) with Adidas, drank a Coke. The queens wore elegant patterned silk *kiras* (traditional dress for women) and were gracious yet accessible as they cheerfully poured tea for the hikers at the top of the hill before we descended. Years later, at twenty-five, the crown prince became king, thirty-five years after his father had become the leader of this Buddhist kingdom.

The health assistant let us see the lists of patients who had received free non-scalpel vasectomies. Tshering showed us the safe home delivery kits she provided to mothers who chose to deliver at home and correctly recited how she managed the different complications in labour and delivery about which we questioned her.

"But only half the women come for prenatal care. The homes are far. It is many hours' walk to our BHU, but before this was built, it was many days away from most families. Ninety percent of women are now within a three-hour walk of a BHU, but if a woman feels well, why should she come? She has so much to do — farming, cooking, looking after her family. But she knows we are here when she goes into labour. She can send a runner to get us. All of us would be proud to walk to her home to deliver her. We have all been trained. We have medicines to control bleeding and convulsions. We know we can send her to the district hospital if there are problems, and she needs more help than we can provide. We are moving, but we have a long way to go. There are only four facilities in the whole country that can do emergency Caesarean sections out of twenty-five hospitals.[15] In two more years this will be doubled. We are walking steadily on the road. Before, these were only dreams."

After meeting Pema and her baby, we talked late into the night with Tshering and her colleagues, hearing their ideas on how health care could be improved, how they needed better transportation for women with difficult deliveries, how distressed they were that a woman had died the week before from an obstructed labour, how far they had to travel to reach the next level of care.

I arrived unexpectedly in the villages where there were health facilities to visit. Still, people found places for us to sleep. In another village I was given one whole three-bedroom house to share with a team from UNICEF. Its owners had travelled to a sacred ceremony at a monastery farther east and were honoured to have their home used by us. Blankets, still in their plastic packets from China and waiting to be sold in the market, were lent to us for warmth for the night and returned to their packets and the market stall in the morning. Red rice with green chilies, strong cheese, and fatty pork were cooked at a neighbour's home and brought to us in large metal pans.

As I journeyed east, I found a small village with a restaurant where a slight, apple-cheeked woman welcomed strangers to her home and kitchen. I made polite conversation as I checked out her four husbands, discovering polyandry for the first time. She explained that each husband had his strengths: one was good at marketing, one at cooking, one made her laugh, and one she gazed at fondly and blushed. The woman cooked over a wood fire, and the room was cozy and warm, with pillows covered in handwoven cloth to sit up against.

I talked with the woman who was also a weaver. I have two looms in my northern Ontario home, so I was happy to share techniques, and I selected some of her fabric to take back to Canada. I wanted to have a piece of this country to comfort me when I returned home. I wanted to look at the woven cushions in their distinctive red, blue, and green patterns and remember this time. I realized how blessed I was to be here, planning to continue to improve the quality of health care through better trained and supported health workers, to continue to address maternal mortality and the slowly emerging HIV epidemic, and to strengthen the work with the monks, who were an important part of the water and sanitation effort.

Three weeks later I returned to Thimphu. I called my Canadian friend Anne Currie, who had lived in Bhutan for years and had a Bhutanese family. She came over to Hotel Druk for tea. Anne had first arrived in Bhutan as a teacher, following Father Mackey's tradition of helping to establish schools in remote areas.

"So what do you think?" she asked me as she juggled Jessie, her daughter, in her arms. "Aren't you just in love with Bhutan?"

I tried to explain. "It's more complicated. Everything is integrated — health, spirituality, the commitment of Buddhism, and the royal family. It's like everything is growing in a holistic way for positive changes. There's leadership for health." I picked up the book she had lent me about Father Mackey. "I think I get this now, where he writes, 'I am convinced of the real presence of the Spirit in Hinduism and Buddhism. It is very much alive in the peasant people of Bhutan. Bhutan has taught me how to pray. I had been trying to grasp God with my mind. It can't be done. The ordinary Bhutanese taught me to grasp God with my heart, to experience God in prayer, in every detail of my life and to have greater trust and faith in human nature.'[16]

"Yeah, Anne, I want to be like him. When he says, 'I am a better Jesuit, a better priest, and a better human being because of my years in India and Bhutan.' Did you know he boasted that he had never converted a single Bhutanese to Christianity, claiming they didn't need to be converted with such a strong spirituality? For those who questioned this, he added, 'Many think I am a heretic. However, I am convinced that the Lord loves me. That is all that matters.' Somehow he found flow. He remained himself and he added value, but he let the people lead. They led, but they acknowledged him. The Bhutanese government appointed him honorary adviser to education for life. We need to remember how carefully he walked in balance when we're working and living with other cultures. There are mysterious strengths in culture. We have to find ways to work with those currents when we're making changes for health."

I watch the prayer flags, which I had bought in Thimpu, flying in sight of water to appease the *nagas* — Sanskrit water snake spirits — to keep my family safe in Haileybury, Ontario. I can draw on their strengths and remember to be hopeful when my own spirit is overwhelmed and despairing. My prayers fly on those flags toward the universe: It is possible to improve the health of pregnant women in our lifetime. What needs to be done is known — family planning, midwives to deliver babies safely, and emergency obstetric care when problems develop. The highest level of political commitment is needed to make sure the poor can have access to these services. Reducing these maternal deaths is a collective global responsibility, and there are models to build on such as Bhutan's.

BANGLADESH, 1990–2010
Halida's Daughters, 1990

Halida murmured a steady chant as she stroked the warm forehead of Nasreen, her daughter. Every three or four minutes Nasreen writhed and choked back sobs. This was the second day. Nasreen could barely sip water.

Sometimes instead of clutching her belly, she grabbed her head in both hands and cried, "*Aiee!*"

Halida's younger daughter, Geeta, aged eight, looked up, serious and intent. She had a small ball made of wound rags that she tossed back and forth in her hands. Her *shalwar kameez* was dark red and burgundy, a little ragged, the trousers darker burgundy and the top lighter red, with a burgundy floral pattern at the cuffs, neck, and hem. Her feet were bare. She had already cooked the rice and dahl for the family, and the heavy smell of cooking still hung in the air. The men — her brother and father — were at the mosque but would be back soon. Geeta threw the ball to the rooster, which pecked busily in the corner, and laughed when he jumped back, shrieking. Then she hopped back herself, astonished and puzzled when her mother shouted at her. Her mother never shouted.

"Go ... go and get Zafrullah, the village quack! The baby isn't coming." Geeta skipped outside, kicking the ball along the path beside the rice paddies. The quack wasn't far. She coughed politely outside his hut and waited.

Zafrullah came to the doorway. "Your sister? I am coming."

Geeta was sure it had only been a few minutes, maybe ten, since her mother had sent her to Zafrullah's. But as the young girl and the old man in his white *longhi*, prayer cap, and *dhoti* arrived at Geeta's home, the wailing lament of Halida assaulted their ears before they could enter.

"Aieee! She has been taken by spirits! Her body was shaking, and spit came out of her mouth, and then everything stopped. No breathing." Halida started crying, ragged sobs that shuddered throughout her body. Then she halted and began a murmuring chant as she stroked Nasreen's still-warm forehead.

Halida's Daughters, 2000

Kanti, the sari-clad paramedic with her simple sandals, led me through the green rice paddies along a winding footpath to a one-room hut. A messenger had run anxiously to the small health centre we were visiting, asking us to come quickly to see a young woman who was having a difficult birth. We poked our heads into the dark room, only a little light issuing through a curtained window and the doorway. Inside, four Bangladeshi women crowded around a wooden pallet on which a young pregnant woman, Geeta, maybe eighteen years old, lay writhing in pain and whimpering. On a shelf above her a rooster crowed in sympathy. Two thin, dark men — father, husband — were outside chewing betel nut and spitting red juice with loud splats.

Inside, the traditional birth attendant, two neighbours, and the girl's mother, Halida, offered Geeta worried advice, stroked her hands, and mopped her brow with cool, wet cloths. They had been struggling to bring this first baby into the world for twenty hours. The room was smoky from the wood fire on which water was boiling. Halida put up a hand to cover her mouth and her eyes so we couldn't see her tears. "No, not this one, too. I have already lost her sister, Nasreen."

The capable family health visitor took a battered blood pressure cuff from a worn bag. Intent on her task, she pursed her lips as she took the blood pressure. Her eyes signalled to me that the reading was high. She pulled a wooden "fetoscope" to her ear, placed it on the swollen belly of the delivering woman, and tried to time the fetal heart, but she couldn't hear a beat through the tense, contracted uterus. Geeta's feet and ankles were swollen. She covered her eyes with her hands and cried in Bangla that she had a pounding headache, which was blurring her vision. Kanti pulled on plastic gloves and discreetly checked how dilated Geeta was. Only a fingertip. We had no medicines for pain, to reduce the blood pressure, or to treat convulsions if this case worsened into toxemia. Unless this baby could be delivered, both Geeta and her child would die.

We all had our roles. The rooster was still crowing. The traditional birth attendant had recognized the need for backup and had sent the neighbour for help. Kanti, the paramedic, had now decided to transfer the young woman. She knew there were medicines and doctors available at the Upazila Health Complex or, if surgery was needed, at one of two district hospitals farther away. The worried, murmuring women supported Geeta on a personal level, and the men in the family were busy collecting money to help pay any costs.

Two district hospitals for complicated referrals were available, each four hours away by road and ferry if we provided a vehicle. We sent a message by runner to the next health centre for our Jeep to return and prepared Geeta for a rickshaw wagon ride along the rice paddy path to meet our vehicle on the main road. When we got to the Jeep, we crowded in, making room for the labouring girl, her mother, the paramedic, the traditional birth attendant, and cloth-covered baskets of food and garments. We opted for the hospital we had seen the day before, since we knew it had good resources: an obstetrician-gynecologist who could do a Caesarean section if necessary, a pediatrician, and anaesthesia. They had only been trained and posted there the previous year.

When we arrived, the specialist team helped us move Geeta out of the Jeep. The obstetrician-gynecologist could hear a fetal heartbeat. She sedated the teenager and gave her oxygen, painkillers, and drugs to lower her blood pressure.

I was now working for CIDA and the World Bank, assessing how best to improve maternal health. We were evaluating the quality of care available at all levels — village aid posts, rudimentary clinics, cottage hospitals, referral centres. This was my tenth visit to Bangladesh, this time in a different area from Chittagong.

We carried on in the Jeep to finish our visits to the other clinics, six hours delayed. The visits that day had to be shortened, but the villagers had been waiting so long for us that we couldn't disappoint them. At each stop we explained why we had been delayed. Finally, very late in the day, as the purple dusk settled, we returned to the city centre. On the shore of a holy lake by a temple with wide pavilions, we met the rest of our health appraisal team, which had visited different communities. Bangladeshi families strolled peacefully along the shoreline. The mayor and chief medical officer came to greet us, telling us that the woman we had brought in had delivered a healthy baby boy. The family was giving out sweets and celebrating — *Alhamdulillah!* Praise be to Allah!

After our arrival back in Dhaka, we discovered that Geeta's story had already spread among humanitarian and health workers and the government. It was an unusual tale in a country where only one-third of the women had even one prenatal visit, 90 percent delivered at home, and hospitals were only beginning to be seen as places that cared for women risking death to bring life into the world. But in places where female paramedics, supported by the governments of Bangladesh and their development partners, had been increasingly caring for pregnant women and their children, there had been a continuing decrease in the deaths of women during labour and delivery.

———————

The challenges of maternal health in Bangladesh were very different from those in Bhutan. Yet both countries were achieving progress, both had mostly home deliveries, both had made mother-and-child health a national priority, both had mobilized money from other countries to help, and both were trying to improve their health system, making skilled attendants at delivery and emergency obstetric care more available to poor women.

Two days after our experience with Geeta, we were in the northeastern region of the country, about two and a half hours by road from Sylhet Medical College Hospital. We had seen the facilities at this teaching hospital the day before. We were now visiting a district hospital; we had just seen the Mother and Child Welfare Centre in the same town. Both were capable of Caesarean sections and other emergency obstetric care services. We were in the noisy, dirty casualty department. Forty or so patients were crowded on the floor. One was a woman in labour, whose mouth was full of froth and whose unseeing eyes were turned upward. Her chest heaved with rapid, ragged breaths, and her pulse fluttered wildly at her neck. She had an intravenous drip with magnesium sulfate running.

I recalled years earlier when none of the hospitals were equipped to manage pre-eclampsia/toxemia, and how hard we fought to get the money, training, and staff to manage obstetric complications in hospitals. It had taken years to get magnesium sulfate (the drug of choice to treat pre-eclampsia/toxemia) accredited on the essential drugs list. This is the simplest and most effective treatment to save women's lives from a complication in pregnancy that leads to convulsions and death from toxemia. For bureaucratic reasons the government had forbidden its use, even though this was the standard of care recommended by the World Health Organization.

Female relatives held each wrist of the woman in labour. They stroked her hands and said calming words. I asked Dr. Shirin to translate. "We have travelled with our sister for twelve hours. We came by boat, by rickshaw. She has been convulsing for the past eight hours. But the doctors here tell us they are afraid to do a Caesarean section. They do not know what to do, she is so sick. They say she has to go to the Sylhet Medical College Hospital, but we have no money for the ambulance. The ambulance for this hospital is busy on another call, and the private ambulance is very expensive."

Furious, I turned to my colleagues from the Mother and Child Welfare Centre (MCWC). Their facility was on the family planning side of the health ministry. The district hospital was with the health directorate. Health care in Bangladesh was provided in these two separate jurisdictions. In the early days of independence, donors had pushed to promote family planning and had created a strong department just for that. Health had come second. Decades later the same donors had realized that to support the health of pregnant women, co-operation between these departments was necessary, so they had tried to force integration, which the government had refused since that would have affected seniority and salaries in the two departments if they were amalgamated.[17]

Somewhat forcefully, I asked Dr. Mizan, my Bangladeshi counterpart on the team and the liaison with the head of the MCWC, if transport could be arranged.

"Yes, for half of the price of the private ambulance," he said.

"Well, have them get it organized and make it available for this patient. The MCWC should have offered to co-operate before." I dug into my purse and gave the money to Dr. Mizan. "We may be too late, but we have to try." The family had done its part. They had recognized there was a problem, but they'd had delays in transportation to get to the facility, and now the care they needed wasn't available. We knew it would take them nearly three hours to get to Sylhet, where a C-section could be performed. But at least the patient would have magnesium sulfate while she was travelling. That was more than she would have had ten years ago.

The two women on the floor began a steady murmuring prayer chant as they stroked the forehead of their sister. They would keep praying. She still had a chance to survive.

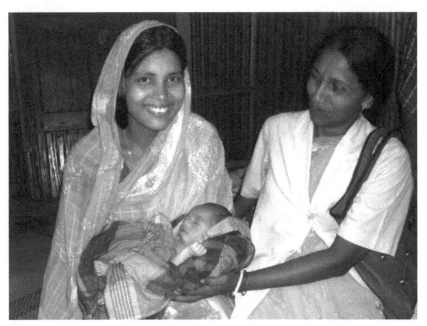

A skilled community birth attendant in Bangladesh does a post-partum check the day after she safely delivered this woman's baby at home.

In the three decades that I have worked in Bangladesh, starting in 1990, maternal health has steadily improved. Family planning is a high priority and is used by half the women in the country. Access to legal abortion is easy (by renaming the procedure "menstrual regulation"; "abortion" is illegal). Very slowly, emergency obstetric care is improving, and efforts are being made to allow poor women access to that care by training general practitioners to do C-sections and anaesthesia. Skilled birth attendants in communities are being trained, similar to the model developed in Indonesia linking poor delivering women with low-cost care in their homes, as well as assisting referral when things go wrong.

In 2001 the external review of the health sector noted that maternal health was further off track than the impressive 40 percent drops in children's deaths. And the government of Bangladesh responded to the challenge: Dr. Jahir Uddin Ahmed, the head of maternal health and family planning for the government of Bangladesh, agreed with our findings and requested me as external technical assistance to help them facilitate the development of a maternal health strategy. This developed training for community-based skilled birth attendants, who could do safe home births, and also provide a link to emergency obstetric care providers.

Between 2001 and 2010, the maternal mortality ratio (MMR) declined from 322 to 194 per 100,000 live births. Seeking facility-based care for maternal complications increased from 29 percent to 46 percent between 2001 and 2010. Since 2010 the MMR has stalled. Over 50 percent of deliveries still occur at home. Only 40 percent of facilities have supplies of injectable oxytocin to stop hemorrhage and only 28 percent have injectable magnesium sulphate to treat eclampsia. The Caesarean section rate at 31 percent is twice the recommended WHO norm for emergency obstetric care. Less than 40 percent of facilities have 24/7 skilled birth attendants and only 3 percent are ready with staff, drugs, and equipment to provide maternal care. Hemorrhage and eclampsia account for 55 percent of maternal deaths. Less than 50 percent of health-care providers at Upazila (district) and 20 percent of private hospitals have someone trained in emergency obstetric care. While progress has been made, supplies, staff, and equipment are still not available where and when needed.[18]

ZAMBIA, 2001

One of the challenges of foreign aid is the need to get money to the places where it is needed to save the lives of vulnerable mothers, their children, and people living with illnesses such as HIV/AIDS. To plan a large support funded by several European and other donors to the health sector in Zambia, I was a team member, together with Jens and David Porter. We were part of the new vogue, the sector-wide approaches where all the development partners pool their money into the government pot, thereby replacing less coordinated individual projects run by different donor countries, each with their own implementing teams. But Zambia at the time was a country beset by corruption, increasing the difficulty of designing health sector supports to reduce the deaths of pregnant women and other vulnerable groups.

Our team leader was Leo Deville, whom Jens knew well and with whom I had worked in Zimbabwe. There was an air of fun and festivity as we reconnected. After taking a few moments to get comfortable with each other, Jens and David made plans to visit the warehouse, which was the central medical store in Lusaka, Zambia's capital. Their aim was to review the distribution of essential drugs. In most developing countries the system for procuring and distributing drugs is often very corrupt, since large amounts of money can be made by embezzling drugs and selling them on the black market. This includes medicines that have been ordered to save the lives of pregnant women. So, within a team, different experts see different aspects of a situation, including the varying roles played by corrupt senior officials. Within a team it is important to share these perspectives. As our assignment progressed, and in the subsequent years, we began to see clearly two sides of a coin. On one side lies the importance of foreign aid in improving health outcomes; on the other is the debilitating corruption of the systems through which money is delivered to a developing country.

I was responsible for the evaluation of sexual and reproductive health, which included an assessment of maternal and child health and HIV/AIDS. I first visited Kitwe (the second largest city in Zambia), then arrived in Ndola, the third largest city in Zambia and home to the largest hospital in the Copperbelt. The Copperbelt Province is mineral-rich but had higher rates of HIV — an unhappy consequence of mining, which had boosted Zambia's economy until the price of copper fell. The medical superintendent reported terrible shortages of drugs, empty government trucks from the essential drugs program passing by the hospitals, delivering nothing or dropping off meagre packages of bandages.

Jens was interested in the stories I had told him about these empty trucks passing by hospitals. In his first preliminary visit to the drugs warehouse with David Porter, Jens had already seen the shipments of HIV drugs and supplies financed by the World Bank: one, the bills of lading were stamped in the warehouse showing they had been officially received; two, the containers turned out to be empty; three, donors had been complaining for several years about misappropriation of funds by the permanent secretary (PS) of health, which included selling drugs on the black market; and four, the proceeds of that embezzlement were shared with President Chiluba who, not surprisingly, had refused to sack the PS. Jens requested a more detailed site visit to the essential drugs warehouse in the capital.

"Not possible," he was told.

More requests went up the chain of command. The president and the minister of health finally gave permission. Jens and David arrived to find a well-stocked warehouse as well as a logistics area staffed with armed guards and brand new, brightly painted trucks. The two men stepped cautiously inside the building where they were subjected to a rough external body search by a uniformed guard. The guard led them to a counter where they were photographed and fingerprinted. Jens and David caught each other's eye with mounting anxiety. This had never happened before in a technical visit to an essential drugs warehouse.

Jens pointed to a huge screen on the wall. "What's that?" he asked the guard. The guard refused to respond. Jens raised a questioning eyebrow at David. They were looking at a computerized map that used a global positioning system to track all the trucks and their exact whereabouts. Jens and David noted that Angola seemed to feature prominently in the distribution system, as did the Democratic Republic of the Congo.

What, besides drugs, could be transported across Zambia from Angola? How did the Democratic Republic of the Congo fit in? Jens had done some research before coming to Zambia. He had discovered that the essential drugs program was being run by a company on a government contract. The company had links to the arms trade and the South African diamond market.

———

I arrived at the maternity block. Sixty pregnant women sat patiently in the waiting area for their antenatal check. They had already been waiting for two hours, and more women were streaming in through the doors, most carrying babies on their backs. Although prenatal care could be provided in a smaller health centre, these women all lived near the hospital. Here they could also be tested for HIV, which couldn't be done in smaller centres yet. The drug room still had contraceptives, though supplies were short for injectable Depo-Provera. There were no anti-malarials to treat or prevent malaria for the pregnant women at higher risk for the disease.

The nurse-midwife in charge saw the women one at a time, trying to impart a little sense of privacy, though her examining room was close to the waiting area, and her voice was slightly audible as a murmur. She had a stained, crumpled, unlabelled box on her desk with condoms, which she offered to each woman. Although these women were pregnant, the nurse-midwife, Naailah, explained discreetly to them that they still needed to be protected from any illnesses that could be sexually transmitted. Naailah wished she could check each woman for syphilis, but the Rapid Plasma Reagin (RPR) test kits to check for syphilis had run out months ago. She knew that about a third of the women she was seeing were HIV positive, but nevirapine to protect their babies from infection had also been stocked out.

Naailah was exhausted, and sweat already dripped off her forehead, darkening the underarms on her uniform, even though it was still morning. She had worked a double shift on the labour ward and was now doing prenatals. Naailah hadn't slept for thirty hours, and she still had a long day ahead. Three of her friends on the labour ward were off sick, so she had worked to cover their shifts. No one wanted to talk about the fact that they, too, probably had HIV — they were steadily losing weight, and there were no anti-retroviral drugs available. And no new health workers could be hired. Under the guidance of the International Monetary Fund and the World Bank, poor countries such as Zambia had been forced to lay health workers off to save money so debts (to richer countries) could be repaid.[19] There simply weren't enough health workers, and the ones who did work weren't paid a living wage, which meant that everyone had to moonlight with a private practice or another business in order to feed their families, leading to a high absentee rate. Health workers were busy at other jobs earning money, at home taking care of ill family members, or were sick themselves.

David and Jens decided to bury their fears. How would it help the poor communities if the obvious distortion of the essential drugs program was explained to the European governments we were working for?

Jens said to me angrily, "Somehow we have to get money down to the ground. Somehow we have to bypass seriously corrupt systems. Somehow we have to hope that the Zambians themselves will rid themselves of evil leaders. You know what they say here? 'When two elephants fight, it is the grass that gets broken.' Remember what happened the last time donors complained to Chiluba about the PS? The donors cut off the money, and it had a devastating impact on the poor people here in Zambia. And the donors couldn't get their act together, either. Remember that meeting when the Japanese were so forgiving of the politicians? 'Of course,' they said. 'Leaders at the top steal. We know this from our own country.' Or the Swedes who initially challenged the government and then backed down? Remember, Gretchen, when we taught you to say to SIDA [Swedish International Development Agency] in bad Swedish — 'You are just hypocrites'?"

I moved on to the labour ward. Namwene had arrived at the hospital bleeding, probably a placenta previa. She had lost at least two pints of blood and was shocky. Her dark skin was almost pale. Quickly, she was typed and cross-matched and transfusions were prepared, the theatre was made ready, and a general duty doctor was located who could do the Caesarean section, with a nurse available to give the anaesthetic. Both the nurse and doctor had been working for more than twenty-five hours. They joked as they pushed the patient's bed, squeaking on its rusty, slightly bent wheels, over worn green linoleum into the theatre.

Leaving them, I went on by Jeep to a mission hospital to meet with families struggling to care for their HIV-positive relatives with help from the Catholic home-based care program. The families were desperately poor, and there were few dressings and little supplemental food. They had no plastic or rubber sheets for the chronic diarrhea of their family members, and the caregivers, mostly women, were exhausted. The mission hospital was trying to appeal to churches abroad for help, but funding was down. There had been a cholera epidemic in the city, and the HIV-positive patients were at greater risk; many of them had already died. One family we met had lost three HIV-positive adult children to cholera.

———◆———

David and Jens tried various versions of a way to ensure that minimal funds went to the corrupt essential drugs program run by the government. Medicines were crucial to support midwives and to assist with emergency obstetric care. But the drugs and equipment had to reach the people who needed them. The team took evening walks to discuss what would and could be said, debating as we wandered along a muddy path through a field filled with bluebirds nesting in deep reddish-brown shrubs.

Jens advised, "There's excellent potential for a system run by the Churches' Health Association of Zambia. Without directly accusing the government of corruption, why don't we write something like this? 'For drugs and medical supplies, a parallel storage and distribution system should be developed using mission facilities rather than government. Transport for monthly distribution of consolidated deliveries to districts and hospitals should be subcontracted to local haulage companies, and the potential benefits of competition in the supply system should be investigated.'"[20]

The team agreed on the wording, designed to avoid the corrupt systems and be implemented as a model of "public-private partnership." Nothing was said about the corruption.

———◆———

I was still at the mission hospital. One girl who was HIV positive was fourteen. She was pregnant, and her HIV status was discovered in her prenatal visit. I quietly asked the nun in charge what her story was.

"The family had no money for school fees," I was told. "She seems to have had sex with her uncle. He was helping the family with money. The uncle and his wife are also HIV positive. She is young, and she is at higher risk of dying in pregnancy. But HIV will get her soon in any case. We have so few patients on ARVs [anti-retroviral drugs]."

———◆———

In 2007 former President Chiluba was found guilty of stealing $46 million of public money by a U.K. court with the support of Zambian authorities who provided information.[21] A Lusaka magistrate sentenced the former permanent secretary of health to five years of hard labour for his corruption and embezzlement charges. In 2007, on an assignment in Papua New Guinea, I met one of his prosecutors, who had received death threats and who had courageously struggled on with the support of his wife, a doctor who specialized in HIV/AIDS.

The anti-corruption sweep also targeted one of the former ministers of health, an articulate and intelligent man whom we donors had adored, never dreaming how much he would ultimately steal. He had successfully evaded capture by hiding in an underground cavern, accompanied by a box painted to look like a computer, complete with "electronic attachments" that warned him of search parties. The former minister of health was found, according to legend, when an army captain asked a traditional healer for advice in order to capture this fugitive. The healer had explained that the troops would have to remove their underpants in order to avoid detection by some type of computerized tracking system that the healer had seen in his vision next to the fugitive, who was hiding underground. The troops had followed the directions given to them by the traditional healer to the hiding place. In a daring raid, the soldiers had removed their underpants and had found this senior official.

In May 2009 the health sector was again hit with scandal. Two million dollars (U.S.) had been embezzled, some from the sector-wide pool, or basket fund, and some from the Global Fund to Fight AIDS, Tuberculosis, and Malaria.[22] A whistleblower called the Anti-Corruption Commission, which was investigating. Funds from the Swedish and Dutch governments to the health sector were frozen. Over half of the funding to the health sector normally came from donors. Wide international support was given to the Zambian economist Dambisa Moyo, educated at both Oxford University and Harvard, who argued in her book *Dead Aid* that development aid encouraged corruption.[23] While some money from our development assistance was embezzled, there had been huge progress at saving the lives of pregnant women. And if almost half of the money in the health sector came from foreign aid, this was an important achievement of those funds.

The Zambian 2007 Demographic and Health Survey (DHS), which is done every five years, showed a 30 percent drop in deaths of children under five since the previous survey. The deaths of pregnant women dropped 60 percent, from 729 to 449 per 100,000 live births. Ninety-four percent of women received antenatal care, and nearly 50 percent of deliveries occurred in health facilities. HIV positivity had stabilized at fewer than 15 percent. Since 1992, contraceptive use has more than doubled to over 50 percent. The availability of anti-retroviral drugs has more than doubled.[24]

Does foreign aid fuel corruption? *Nchekeleko* — give me my share, cut me a slice! Or is foreign aid an important contribution to improving health outcomes? In 2012 the European Union, building on the momentum in improving maternal health, committed a potential €44 million in additional funds to accelerate progress in reducing HIV and maternal and child mortality in Zambia. Progress has continued. By 2014, the total fertility rate had dropped to 5.3 from 6.2 in 2007. But the percentage of teenaged pregnancies has hardly changed in the last six years. Nearly 45 percent of women in union use modern contraceptives in 2014 compared to only one in three women in 2007. Infant mortality and under-five mortality have declined by 58 percent and 61 percent, respectively, over the last two decades. Sixty percent of infants are fully immunized by age one. Half of the population has access to an insecticide treated bed net to prevent malaria. Over 80 percent of mothers with a birth in the five years preceding the survey were protected against neonatal tetanus, and two-thirds of women had skilled attendants at delivery. HIV prevalence had dropped from 16 percent to 13 percent from 2000 to 2014.[25,26]

TANZANIA, 1997–2006

The road stretched empty ahead and behind our pickup truck. This was a very remote and rural area of Tanzania, a few hours north of a town called Songea, in the Ruvuma region of southeastern Tanzania. A man with a bicycle was desperately trying to flag us down. On the back of the bike was a basket, and in the basket, his pregnant wife. He was taking her to hospital, a trip that could take four hours even without a pregnant woman in the basket and probably double that given her current condition. Labour was well underway.

My Tanzanian colleagues from the national Planned Parenthood affiliate and I stopped to offer help. In her one antenatal check, when she was four and a half months pregnant, she had been advised to have this baby in the hospital because this was her sixth delivery with higher risks of hemorrhage. When her contractions began five hours earlier, she had sent a messenger to find her husband on the family farm, but it took all that time for him to leave his work and obtain a bicycle on which to carry her. The husband had to accompany her in order to pay for her care at the hospital.

Standing beside the bike, with a toothless face wreathed in smiles, was the labouring woman's mother. We offered to transport the family. My colleagues moved from their seat to the open back of the truck, joining the community-based distributors (who dispense contraceptives in their villages), the husband, and his bike. The mother-to-be and her mother moved onto the bench seat, the older woman with a bag of worn metal pots and well-washed rags.

I asked, through the driver who acted as translator, how long the woman had been in labour and how many times she had given birth. Did the grandmother know how to deliver? What did she have available for the delivery? She pointed proudly to the clean patterned cotton rags torn from *kangas*, or long skirts, and the small, battered tin pots. She had brought no water, but we had several plastic bottles of it. The labouring woman was silent and then gave a small, worried sigh.

Turning around, I lifted the pregnant woman's skirt to see the baby's head crowning, as well as meconium (fetal bowel movement) staining, which indicated fetal distress. I took one of our bottles of water, poured it over my hands, and crossed myself, as did the smiling grandmother. Then I carefully protected the baby's head as it emerged, glistening, the dark hair wet and streaked with its mother's blood-tinged mucus. Holding the baby's head with my open left hand, I slowed its arrival and tucked the fingers of my right hand to feel around the neck. The cord was wrapped around the baby's neck twice. Still twisted in my seat, I untangled the cord and delivered the baby boy while we were driving. The blue-faced infant didn't cry despite my desperate efforts to spank him into some kind of response.

Seconds later a small health centre miraculously came into view on the right-hand side of the road. I asked the driver to run for a midwife and tell her we had a newly delivered, unresponsive baby in the truck.

Out came the smiling Tanzanian midwife, wearing a starched white uniform and a blue-banded hat. She pulled on gloves and carried a metal basin and a syringe to suction the mucus from the baby's mouth and nose. The midwife managed to get the baby to cry lustily before she delivered the placenta, the afterbirth. Moments later we were helping mother, child, and grandmother into the little clinic. I was relieved. We would all be safe now. This mother and her newborn would be in good hands, and I could depart without worries.

The midwife was more concerned about the mess in our pickup truck and wanted to go outside to clean it. "No problem!" I cried. So the midwife took the newborn boy and placed him, naked and uncovered, on a bare metal weighing scale. She then laid this newly delivered woman on the concrete floor, took a hose connected to the local water tank, and washed her down with cold water, cleaning the blood from her legs, genitals, and abdomen. I washed my hands with iodine soap, remembering that HIV positivity in people aged fifteen to forty-nine was about 7 percent in that area, and I had delivered the baby with no gloves!

If that open, untravelled road hadn't brought our unlikely pickup truck, would this baby boy have lived or been strangled on that cord during his birth?

While there have been notable improvements in maternal health in Bangladesh, Nepal, Indonesia, China, and Bhutan, despite the challenges of distance, the same geographic hurdles and poorly functioning health systems have made it harder for these same improvements in Africa. There are still too many hours that separate families from the essential care they need during labour and delivery, hours that can easily lead to the deaths of a mother and a baby — unless chance intervenes.

In 2006, almost ten years after my first visit, Tanzania was far ahead of its targets on infant mortality; the deaths of children were falling: down by 40 percent in the past five years. But for pregnant women the picture was still grim. Nearly 70 percent of women with no education delivered at home, and just over 1 percent of them had access to a Caesarean section.[27] Over 60 percent of women in Tanzania reported they couldn't get someone with midwifery skills to deliver their babies and provide emergency care when things went wrong.[28] The barriers included lack of money because of user fees, lack of transport, or the distance to a health facility.[29] In short, the deaths of pregnant women were up. But the action of the government, supported by its partners, has started to turn this situation around.[30]

I was sitting with Professor "Prof" Hiza, a highly esteemed Tanzanian physician and academic, on the slightly brown grass under a tree with a huge protective canopy in front of a hut. Wind rustled the leaves in the tree, making them crackle. It had been a three-hour drive on rough, rutted roads, followed by a half-hour walk down a muddy path, to get to this Maasai village. The *enkang*, or barrier, surrounding the loaf-shaped mud-and-cow-dung hut was made of acacia bushes. I was the team leader of the external review of the health sector, an independent group of experts reporting to the Tanzanian government, various donor countries, NGOs, and the United Nations. This assignment involved visiting different communities and health facilities, as well as comparing statistics on achievements in health. We would then present our findings to a mix of Tanzanians in government and non-governmental organizations as well as representatives of the *wazungu* (Swahili for "expatriate") donors to Tanzania.

Prof and I were listening to Neema, who was shyly not quite meeting our eyes as she explained how she had given birth to her daughter. Her earlobes were adorned with heavy beaded rings, leaving wide, gaping, disc-shaped holes in her ears. A large white necklace ruff accented with blue and yellow beads circled her neck, while a burgundy shawl covered her upper body and breasts over a bright navy blue wrap. Her skin glistened with the sheen of sweat, which gave off an earthy, slightly sweet smell and melded with a wafting suggestion of breast milk. These smells blended with the woodsmoke from the fire she was cooking over. Flies buzzed above our heads, darting to the pot cooking on the fire. Neema's baby was kept close to her body in a sling. Prof translated.

"I was married at thirteen. It was the harvest season. I was chosen at the *emasho* by a *moran* [ceremony to choose a woman in marriage when the *morani*, or newly circumcised warriors, select a bride]. After I was chosen, I was circumcised. I was worth many cows! My father was happy. My husband is a good man, but I barely knew him. I had to leave school to marry. I became pregnant right away and then learned from the women in the village how to be brave when I brought her into the world. The men had to leave. My mother and sisters helped me. They massaged my belly with oil. They boiled the water over this fire. It was late at night, and I could watch the stars high above me through the doorway. I was safe. *Meishoo iyiook enkai inkishu o-nkera* [May the Creator give us cattle and children]."

Prof moved closer to Neema, but he was still turned slightly away from her out of politeness. He asked her difficult questions in a gentle manner over the next hour, waiting respectively for her unpressured responses. "Do you know anyone who has had trouble giving birth? Has anyone you know from this village had to go to the hospital to deliver their babies? Did you know that the circumcision you had, the 'female genital cutting,' makes you more at risk for getting HIV/AIDS or for bleeding giving birth?"

"You have some strange ideas," Neema said. "Once we are betrothed, we are cut. We are brave to face this. My mother paid ten thousand Tanzanian shillings for me to have this done so I would be clean for my husband. And to give birth in a hospital? We couldn't do this. The distance is far. I don't have the money! I wouldn't know where to go. But there is no need. We can manage safely in the village. I had many women with me who knew what to do. Look around you! Look at all these kids playing and laughing. They were all born here. And it was night when my daughter was born. It isn't safe to travel at night." Neema lowered her head and her voice and whispered, "Spirits."

Neema felt supported to give birth in her home village with her family around her and a traditional birth attendant helping her by massaging her contracting belly with oil. Until the health system is sensitive to the emotional and spiritual needs of delivering women, we can't hope to get women who can't afford our care to deliver in a "safer" environment that feels foreign to them.

We returned to the Tanzanian capital Dar es Salaam, "the House of Peace." The other teams I was supervising, which had visited other parts of the country, had similar stories. Less than half of the women in the country had skilled personnel at birth, and that was worsening, not improving, and there was no decrease in the number of babies each woman had — nearly six children each. The mood was angry. I had worked with one colleague in Malawi and Bangladesh before this — Jaap Hamel, who was in a stormy mood. "I lived here for years," he told me. "I speak Swahili. Things are worse than in my time. We have to come down hard."

There were three Tanzanians on the team, and we didn't want to put them in an awkward place. Prof was the eldest and was well-respected by the government and the donors. "We aren't pulling our punches, Gretchen. We are your Maasai warriors. We will protect you when you do the presentation."

We prepared our report. I did some dry runs with colleagues I knew well. They were *wazungu* who had lived in Tanzania for years. On the government side I met with Faustin Njau, who informally supported me. "Stick to your guns," he said. "We know you. You've been coming here for ten years. You and Jens Hasfeldt helped to put our whole sector-wide approach, or basket fund together. You and Jens worked with Mr. Munumbu on that before he was murdered, probably for challenging corruption. We remember when Danida cut off aid to the health sector; you continued working for us even when we forbade you to debrief with the Danish Embassy. We trust you. We will back you."

The development partners weren't so sure. I was told, discreetly, that there would be no need for me to present the team's findings at the Annual Health Summit, where the team leader of the external review always presented the group's report. The team persevered.

A long and complex geographic and emotional journey later, I was called up to a stage to do a presentation summarizing our report. Faustin Njau caught my eye and winked.[31] I congratulated Tanzania on the dramatic improvements in child mortality reduction but cautioned about the need to change strategy to help address maternal health. I finished speaking and stood quietly for a moment. The permanent secretary of health, a woman, spoke out clearly. "We would like a second round of applause for Dr. Roedde. We are prepared to move on maternal health, but we need the support of our partners."

Countries are prepared to act on maternal health. If they are leading, as in Tanzania, we have a coherent framework to support financially.

The air was a brilliant pulsating blue as I emerged into the blasting tropical sun after the presentation. Huge palm trees waved at me. The Indian Ocean pounded the shore, sending up huge, thundering sprays of water. I passed a spear-carrying Maasai warrior, tall in his burgundy robes. He was guarding BMW and Mercedes-Benz cars instead of his customary cattle. Both of us, our cultures, were changing each other.

PAPUA NEW GUINEA, 2006–2008

Tanzania was prepared to act to address worsening maternal mortality, but its government didn't have the money to build stronger health systems to improve maternal health. Other countries that ostensibly had the means, such as oil-rich Nigeria and wealthy, donor-rich Papua New Guinea (PNG), saw increases in the deaths of pregnant women. In PNG, workers had become increasingly frustrated; they knew money was pouring in from countries such as Australia and New Zealand and that money was being made from mining and forestry and other natural resources, but they saw little evidence of what it was accomplishing.

The health-centre staff had gathered and was seated on benches on the porch, having been notified by radiophone the day before that we would be arriving.

The nurse in charge stared at us. "Why are you here? No one has visited this health centre from the provincial administration for two years, and this is the closest and most accessible clinic. We've only had money to do one of our scheduled six outreach patrols in 2006. We know we're not reaching our targets for immunizing children and conducting antenatal clinics. We know if the pregnant women don't meet us on our outreach patrols they won't travel this far by boat when it's their time to deliver."

Stabbing her right index finger sharply at the bowl of lychees and bananas, she continued speaking with anger and frustration. "How do we get

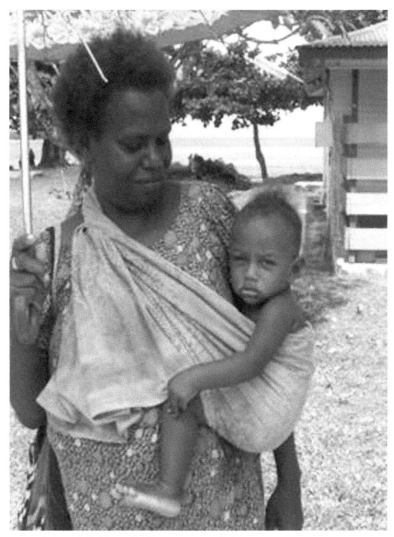

A mother and child in rural Papua New Guinea.

money for fuel for the sterilizer or hurricane lamps for night deliveries? We have to sell fruit to the villagers. No money has come from the government for any of our operating costs. Even our own pay doesn't come regularly."

We looked at her and at one another. I asked with a grim and determined expression, "Haven't you received the extra money from donors and government that's been put aside for support supervision for outreach patrols?"

She shook her head.

I asked if she knew why the money had been increased that was supposed to go to health centres. "Do you know that the death rates of pregnant women have doubled in the past ten years?[32] Do you know there have been no improvements in the numbers of women delivering their babies in health centres?"

I knew the results of the most recent *Demographic and Health Survey*, but no one had bothered to inform health workers so they could try to tackle the problems in the health system. In fact, though the government had declared the situation of maternal deaths a crisis, a largely invisible Ministerial Task Force on Maternal Mortality hadn't yet delivered any practical recommendations. The community health workers who did most of the deliveries in the health centre had no supplies, the outreach patrols that were supposed to visit remote villages to help pregnant women had largely stopped because of lack of money for fuel, and many small aid posts had closed, leaving half of the country with no health care at all.[33]

The nurse in charge shook her head. "How would I learn this? No one comes to talk to us. No one sees how we're getting on. No one gives us any feedback about our work."

———————

Papua New Guinea is an uneasy nation built over thousands of years from eight hundred warring tribal groups and different languages, or *wantoks* (pidgin for "one talk," the concept describes people who speak the same language, an extended clan system), with pidgin the lingua franca. Much of the population lives at subsistence level, while a small elite has become wealthy from timber, fishing rights, sugar and palm oil plantations, oil and gas projects, and vast mineral deposits. This has led to widening inequities in wealth and has contributed to escalating violence.[34]

Mining means money for some, while the majority of the people are unemployed and increasingly angry. Outside the mines the scene is reminiscent of Botswana with its numerous sex workers. Only here the women exchange favours for a betel nut chew and live on a blanket under a tarp. There are areas in PNG that have never seen foreigners, and there are young people who have living grandparents who were cannibals (eating "long pig,"

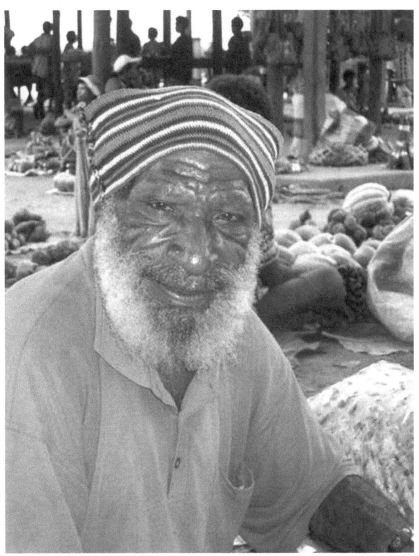

A man in the highlands of Papua New Guinea.

as human flesh was termed). The violence among groups and the vulnerability of women aren't surprising in this context. The number of rapes is going up, as is the rate of HIV infection. Half the health centres are closed, and there are limited outreach patrols. Only half the women in PNG have skilled birth attendants.[35]

As soon as Jens and I boarded our Air Niugini flight, we knew we were in a different culture. Our stewardesses had tattoos — graceful flowers at the corners of their eyes, stars across their foreheads, all in midnight blue ink. One had taken off her shoes to be more comfortable. Already I liked this informal atmosphere. The Papua New Guineans on the plane admired the tattoo of a brown-eyed Susan on my shoulder, while a man from the Cook Islands proudly compared the dark indigo black symbols that covered his arms to my modest flower.

Several hours later, after a stop in the Solomon Islands, we arrived in Papua New Guinea and met the rest of our health-review team. Jens and I were part of a team that was responsible for two independent evaluations every year from 2006 until 2009 of the progress and challenges in the health sector, working on behalf of the government of Papua New Guinea and its development partners, including Australia, New Zealand, and the United Nations.

Two of our colleagues were Australian. Mark was the financial analyst, charged with ensuring the money was flowing to the right priorities. Jo was an expert in organizational development, responsible for human resources management and training. She sported her own tattoo on her back — a complex rendering of a lizard, flowing water, and flowers, courtesy of a South Pacific artist. Later that day we met our PNG counterparts at the National Department of Health (NDOH), who walked barefoot in their offices. Anna Irumai, our main counterpart, greeted us with a hug and a huge, welcoming smile. I had never been anywhere like this before.

Down the hall from Anna Irumai's section was the office of the World Health Organization where we would meet with the UN security adviser. He didn't waste any time alerting us to all the dangers we would face. He counselled us not to walk the stone's throw distance between our hotel and the National Department of Health. To prove his point, he gestured dramatically at the bullet hole in the WHO's boardroom window. The security adviser reminded us that one of the senior WHO advisers had been attacked and nearly killed but was rescued by passersby. He elaborated about another who was driving his car home and was held up in an attempted carjacking. Gunning the engine, the WHO staffer had run over his attackers and escaped.

"This is serious stuff," the UN security adviser continued. "You know there are continuing tribal clashes. When any of these wars are over, each side has payments to make in cash — the *kina* [local currency] bills tucked into long bamboo poles that are carried bravely and presented to the other faction. These huge cash payments can equal thousands of American dollars. How do the tribes get this money in a country with few banks and a yam-based barter system? They call on the *wantok*, the extended family or clan that gives one another jobs and pays for one another's expenses. And the members of the *wantok* based in Port Moresby and other major urban centres can attack affluent citizens or foreigners in order to obtain the needed funds for war reparations. Some money is obtained in this way, hence the violence, including revenge rapes and murders, in the cities."

Betty, the Papua New Guinean UN stress counsellor, added her own warnings. "This is a difficult country. You will be seen as wealthy and with no *wantok* to support you. You are outsiders who don't appear to have any dependents. Anyone living here with paying jobs has to share their salaries with their extended families, as well. The World Health Organization recently shifted the day that their staffers were paid, so it was earlier than the extended family would expect, allowing salaried *wantok* members the chance to put at least some money in the bank before they were obligated to share it. I interviewed all the staff. This was one of two major stresses the national staff faced. The other, among the women, especially when they are pregnant, was being beaten by their husbands."

One of the WHO staffers popped his head into the room we were in. "Don't take them too seriously!" He grinned. "The *wantok* can help expatriates, as well. I am Polish. Once I was attacked by 'rascals' [local term for a criminal] and robbed and left bleeding from knife wounds. I just shouted at them. I reminded them I had a powerful *wantok*. Both nearby hospitals are run by Polish doctors. I told them if they hurt me, in the next war the Polish doctors wouldn't look after their wounded. They aren't stupid. They thought about that for a couple of minutes, spoke among themselves in pidgin, and then bandaged my wounds and transported me, my bicycle, and all my possessions to the nearest Polish-run hospital." Laughing, he left the room.

We listened carefully, but when the security adviser told us not to take taxis, we nodded sagely and then ignored him, choosing instead to use the two taxi companies, Red Dot and Scarlet, deemed safe by the locals since the drivers were accompanied by armed guards at night. We also listened to other technical advisers who worked on behalf of the United Nations and gave us advice on regions we were about to visit. They told us about the head of one of the UN agencies who wanted to travel to a remote area to see how health services were functioning in the rural periphery. His security had to be guaranteed, and a local driver was hired. During the trip, the senior UN adviser engaged the driver in conversation. "So what do you do when you're not picking up work as a driver?"

"I rob and kill people" was his cheerful and honest reply.

Our team had split up to see both high-performing and low-performing areas of the country. Mark and I, together with Yvonne, who was Papua New Guinean, had arrived in this poor province by bush plane. The health indicators here had been terrible though improving slightly in the previous year, with very few women delivering in health centres and many dying on the way to care. We tried to give some encouragement to the frustrated, lychee-stabbing nurse and her staff. We vowed we would go back to the capital and fight harder for direct funding to their health facility.

However, the smooth reply from Permanent Secretary of Health Dr. Nicolas Mann took no responsibility for the fact that no money was getting down to the ground: health centres were closing, outreach patrols had stopped, and pregnant women were dying in increasing numbers. "Quite frankly, you have disappointed me," he said. "I wanted a crisper analysis."

In 2007 we returned to PNG, eager to see if things had improved. I travelled with Dean Shuey, a colleague with the WHO, to Morobe Province, where we met with its provincial health adviser. We asked if he knew the public health priorities of the PNG government. "Of course — immunization, reducing deaths of pregnant women, combating malaria, and attacking HIV/AIDS/TB." He pointed proudly to very nice planning documents, printed and bound, elaborated at great expense with consultation of districts and health centres, outlining the four public health strategic directions. They sat on shelves in his office with carefully numbered and detailed annual activity plans.

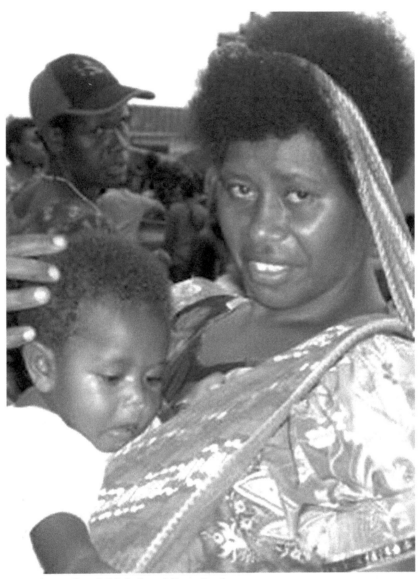

A mother with a child she has delivered at home.

We were curious. "Why then is it that in your province only 40 percent of children are immunized against measles, only 15 percent of women had a supervised delivery, and only 20 percent of women have even one prenatal visit? And the only money being spent to train village birth attendants or to work at the community level is coming from NGOs such as the Salvation Army? Why is it that the church-based facilities that could do outreach so they could actually reach poor women in the communities for antenatal care are funded only to do curative care?"[36]

The provincial health adviser controlled access to much of the money available at the provincial level. Interestingly, we noted the new computer and the new air conditioner humming in his office. We also learned that the meetings to develop the annual activity plans — the same unimplemented plans as the year before — were usually held in very nice hotels over a two-week period, all expenses paid for him and his most senior colleagues. Perhaps this was why there had been little money for these health workers to go out to nearby villages on patrols. Money was spent to plan services for pregnant women; no money was spent to actually implement those plans.

Discouraged, we flew back to Port Moresby and decided to have lunch at a hotel near the airport. We wanted to welcome Jens, who had just arrived after finishing his first round of chemotherapy. Joining us was John, a colleague from the Asian Development Bank. He had been instrumental in setting up this "sector-wide approach" where all donors and government put their money into a common basket to fund mutually agreed priorities.

"It doesn't seem to be working," we complained. "Too much money is getting diverted into administration and isn't helping direct health services."[37]

"You're right," John replied, then suggested we try the curry.

In Papua New Guinea, as in most developing countries, dedicated missionaries provide the majority of health services for the rural poor. We were visiting mission facilities and continuing our review of PNG's health sector. In one mission hospital the nurses were worried. On their outreach patrols to look after pregnant women and their young children in remote villages, they often had to travel with armed guards for protection. Even the mission hospitals faced attack — rape, robbery, and murder. In a country with rising HIV rates, these risks carried an even more serious threat.

Frieda, a nurse-midwife, explained, "We women health workers are provided with HIV drugs for post-exposure prophylaxis — to prevent contracting HIV in the case of rape. Some of us wear female condoms, again to prevent HIV exposure as well as pregnancy in the case of sexual assault. We know that as women we have higher risks of HIV. We are also more likely to be beaten at home or on the road while we are patrolling. But we have to carry on. We have to be brave. We have to serve the women of Papua New Guinea. We know their situation is getting worse and worse. So many die in the villages with no one to look after them when they are pregnant. If we give up as well, if we give in to our own fears, we are just abandoning them."

Our team listened to Frieda and her staff's problems and agreed how difficult it was to do deliveries at night in the dark by candlelight or with a flashlight held in one's mouth. For the very few women who actually came to give birth at the health centre, it was a long walk away from their homes with the risk of rape. There are simple flashlights that can be worn on a band around the head, like a miner's lantern. No one had thought to buy these inexpensive supports to make the lives of midwives easier. In 2017, less than half of births in PNG were attended by midwives, and health facilities were poorly equipped. PNG had a high maternal mortality rate (773/100,000 live births) and a critical shortage of skilled midwives.[38]

We commiserated with them about the cupboards full of expired supplies from 2006, which they hadn't been able to dispose of. Together we wondered why new supplies, contraceptives, and oxytocin to stop bleeding before, during or after delivery, hadn't reached their facilities. They showed us how they had no iron folate to prevent anemia in pregnant women, making it more probable for them to die of hemorrhage. The whole country had been out of stock of this drug for a year. This cheap drug, with limited potential to sell on the black market, had simply not been ordered by government. We promised we would keep on fighting to get them more money and then gave them some from our pockets as encouragement.

As we walked between the two clinic buildings, it was raining heavily, so the staff lent us two umbrellas for the slippery hike down the muddy path. When we travelled back in the boat, the warm rain felt wonderful on the skin. We smiled at one another, even though we were soaked and discouraged.

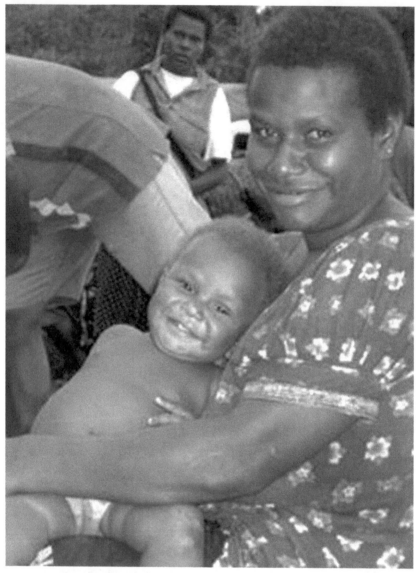

A Papua New Guinean woman with one child in her arms as she watches another child in a garden.

Near the shore, Ruben, the family health coordinator, wisely decided that the narrow footbridge would be treacherous in the rain, so we walked instead across the mudflats to the oyster shell shore on the opposite bank, then up through the village in the rain to our guest house.

A cold shower and change of clothes later, Mark and I headed out for a stroll in what was now a misty grey drizzle. Our path took us past the village green, full of wet, laughing children and adults wearing cheerful team shirts in bright colours — red, yellow, blue. They were playing basketball and soccer on different parts of the field. Down a laneway, there was a garden with a riot of blooming trees, a stilted house at its centre looking out over the wide river to the distant cloudy hills. We waved and smiled at the owner, a woman sitting on the porch watching a toddler run through the garden. Life continued in happy rhythms, seemingly oblivious to the gross government negligence we were seeing. Only one week later this tranquil village was the setting for the local bank manager to give away half a million dollars of the bank's money as ransom to release his kidnapped pregnant daughter.

———————

Planning a schedule took on a whole new rhythm in PNG — more often than not, making any arrangements was linked to the weather. During the rains, it meant we could travel locally by the fast-flowing rivers, but to travel to outlying districts we would have to fly as the downpours made the open seas too treacherous. When the airstrip was inadvertently closed because of a small accident, we were stranded. While waiting to fly to a Catholic hospital, we met Bruce, who worked in education.

"We're facing tough challenges," he said. "Schools are closing because of violence. The elections closed the schools as well as the health-aid posts. Our teachers have been working for months with no salaries, but we have help from the communities that are volunteering labour at the schools. We're struggling with the rising costs, the expense of having to charter planes to fly in examination papers because the airstrips are closing."

We had to agree with Bruce about the rising costs of the airlines, and in our case the concern was the impact this had on health, particularly that of pregnant women. The government had shut down a private air carrier with cheaper services. It now had a monopoly on air service and could charge what it wanted. Airlines refused to carry small packs of vaccines as freight on passenger flights, or to transport a woman needing emergency obstetric care for a subsidized rate. Instead they requested whole planes be chartered at a far higher cost. With the loss of air access many coastal people now faced long voyages on the open sea, and drowning was a constant risk for patients and health workers alike.

In some areas we had discovered the health department had been unable to get delivery of mosquito nets — to protect pregnant women and children under five from malaria — because of the lack of money for shipping by air into the remote communities. So they were still sitting in transit stores after two years. Money from the Global Fund had been disrupted for a number of reasons. The central tender board awarded a contract to an inexperienced supplier who couldn't meet the commitments. The Global Fund stopped the money because the supplier couldn't deliver, and he took the government to court for failing to honour the contract. Politics and corruption added to high costs, and it was the poor who suffered, the poor who couldn't get access to mosquito nets that could save women's and children's lives or afford transport to get to a higher level of emergency obstetric care.

In many ways, however, education was better positioned than health. Every school received money directly to its own bank account, held in trust by the schoolteacher so he or she would have money for limited school supplies. No money was sent directly to the small health centres. The National Department of Health had many excuses. Although the officer in charge of a health centre had similar levels of education to those of a teacher, village committees gave stronger support to schools, volunteering to help the teachers and to ensure that the allocated money was spent wisely.

When it came to health facilities, no one pushed for equal support. Churches allowed their health facilities to receive direct grants, but every time we, as an external independent team, pressed for direct funding of a government health centre, the national government blocked us. It refused even when we backed up our argument with the fact that pregnant women were being charged prohibitive fees for water, or a light source, or simple medicines, which forced women to stay at home and trust their neighbours to assist them through an emergency.

Education was more effective at deploying teachers from local communities in their own areas than health was. Local assistant teachers

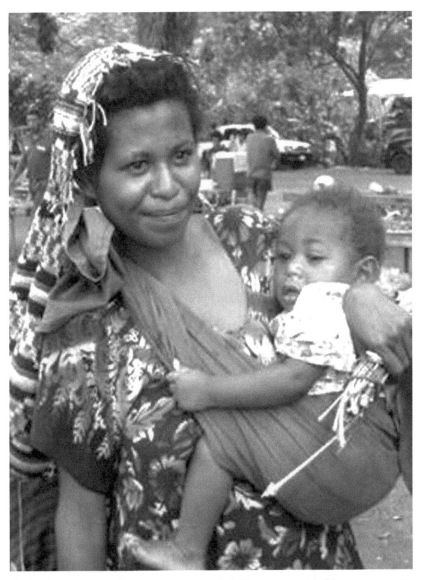

Most of the women who have a supervised delivery are assisted by a community health worker.

from poor, rural PNG communities had been upgraded to fill teachers' posts. In contrast, the health system still seemed dominated by a medical model imported from Australia. Doctors weren't available in the poor rural areas. The "bush doctors," or health extension officers, who were PNG nationals, could only be promoted if they went into administration. So they no longer provided clinical care.

Nurses and midwives frequently had disruptions in their curricula, so there was a backlog to accredit them. Few donor governments were interested in supporting the PNG nationals who were trained as community health workers, the most basic level, and who could deliver babies safely and would accept postings to poor rural areas.

Bruce was the only expatriate — a Brit — who worked with the education team. He proudly described why he had remained in PNG for thirty years. "Such a chance to really make a difference! This isn't a failed state. It is vulnerable. There are important pockets of resilience to build on. I've watched Papua New Guineans take back control of senior positions of leadership, and I'm motivated to see improvement in spite of huge obstacles. We're trying to educate the children, especially the girls. We know this is the future." As I watched him joke with his colleagues in pidgin, I was impressed by his commitment.

When we reached Braun Memorial Hospital, which was supported by the Lutheran Church, in Finschhafen district of the Morobe Province, Leonie, the nurse in charge, greeted us at the gate in her starched white uniform. Leonie looked worried. She told us that the day before one of the outreach patrol nursing teams has been attacked and robbed. Leonie apologized, explaining that when we talked to her staff we would find the nurses upset. They might not want to answer our questions about the hospital and its work.

We offered our condolences in the formal way that seemed expected. Elaborate shows of emotion are frowned upon, since it is simply not possible to dwell on the disasters that continually occur, the ongoing violence.

Touring the hospital, we met with various staff members. The pharmacist on our team inspected the medical store to ensure that essential medicines were available. This faith-based hospital was better supplied, and it managed its stores more efficiently than the government facilities. The staff told us they didn't know they were eligible to receive more government money for upgrading their maternity facilities. They didn't know that this had been written in the provincial annual activity plan with a budget against their hospital's name.

The Dutch Lutheran doctor in charge joined us, apologizing for not feeling well. Three weeks earlier, he had been operating on a possibly HIV-positive patient with a gunshot wound and had received a needle-stick injury. He was still waiting for the results of the patient's HIV test to come back from the central reference lab; the rapid tests were too unreliable. He was on anti-retroviral drugs to prevent infection, but they were making him ill. Nevertheless, he was working twenty-hour days with a small, overworked staff.

Leonie turned and introduced us to another colleague, a Papua New Guinean public health nurse from the provincial administration. "This is Baleb. She is the family health service coordinator."

I looked at her, curious, as I had heard the name years before. "Baleb?"

"Yes."

I asked her if she had ever travelled outside PNG. "Yes, to Liverpool, England, in 1984."

"What did you study?"

"The spring course called Teaching Primary Health Care."

Her name was familiar because she had been a former student of mine from the Liverpool School of Tropical Medicine. Both of us had become rounder with age, desirable in her culture, less so in my own. I had to study her carefully to recognize her face. We reached out our arms and clasped each other on the forearm, warmer than a handshake, not close enough yet for a hug. It had been a quarter century since we had last seen each other. We remembered her story of a midwife in the jungle who had removed, with her bare hands, the retained placenta from a hemorrhaging woman who had just given birth. What *naga*, what snake spirit, had brought us together again?

After our final discussion with the hospital staff, we were taken by ambulance through the small settled area where we finally found a storekeeper willing to reopen his food store. None of us had eaten since early morning, so Baleb and I quickly made hors d'oeuvres, while the owners of the guest house prepared the rest of the dinner. We ate them at a trestle table outdoors under a wooden roof with no walls — nothing to impair our view of the ocean and the stars that had begun to appear. Every now and then Baleb glanced at me. "Twenty-four years since Liverpool!" Then she gazed far into the distance, worriedly thinking about the mother-and-child health team that had been attacked the day before. "Look up!" Baleb said with a slow smile as the Southern Cross came into view in the velvet sky.

The Southern Cross — a new favourite travelling companion when I found myself in countries south of the equator. Have our lives, and the stars, been put in place by something beyond us? I was reminded of my mother's stories of growing up in British Columbia with the Doukhobors, a Russian sect whose name literally means "spirit wrestlers." My own spirit was wrestling with different beliefs as our conversation over dinner drifted into the night: between a faith that life unfolds according to a plan and a conviction that we each must work hard to bring a better world into being.

Jens and I had waited hours for our flight to arrive, and then we were off to Bougainville to continue our assessment on behalf of the PNG government and its humanitarian donors. Bougainville had become a semi-autonomous region after a civil war had erupted in 1989 over control of the Panguna Copper Mine (there are also gold deposits), which was owned by a conglomerate that included Australians. Australia backed the government of Papua New Guinea with an armed response against the rebels in Bougainville, and 10 percent of the population (about 180,000 people) was eventually killed.[39] Peacekeeping forces were withdrawn in 2003, and the area was now considered safe enough to travel in.

To go over to the provincial health office in Buka we had to journey by open boat for ten minutes to a nearby island. Piling into the dinghy, if I closed my eyes I could have been back on Lake Temagami in northern Ontario with Indigenous colleagues and friends driving in open steel boats. The smell of the outboard motor fuel and the growl of the motor took me right back to earlier days seeing patients on the lake. Here, "redskins" is the name given to people from Papua New Guinea, whose skin tone is unlike the dark ebony skin of the people of the North Solomons, also named the Autonomous Region of Bougainville.

It was a tough climb up a long flight of stairs to reach the provincial health office. Jens was struggling to breathe, and we walked slowly, with many rest stops. When we were finally seated at a long conference table, we were astounded by the beautifully organized graphs charting progress in immunization and safe motherhood with detailed comparisons between health centres.

The next day, our trip to reach the region's other major town, Arawa, was even more difficult. The journey took us several bone-crushing hours over deeply rutted roads, including crossing five rivers with no bridges (all had been destroyed in the civil war) and inching our four-wheel-drive hardtop across stony river bottoms with swirling water coming up to the level of the windows.

As we neared the health centre, a barred road off to the right informed us this was the no-go zone. Continued tribal unrest in this area near the closed Panguna Mine was slowly stabilizing, but only outreach workers were allowed into the no-go zone for mother-and-child health patrols. Later we met a nun in full habit who was trying to negotiate a peace settlement.

The burnt-out shell of the old hospital was visible behind prefabricated buildings, which comprised the wards of the health centre that was once a fully functioning hospital. There was no longer a doctor stationed here who could perform essential surgeries such as Caesarean sections. Despite the fact that money in the Health Sector Improvement Program (HSIP) was supposed to be available to transport women for emergency obstetric care, it couldn't be accessed. Instead, a woman was charged five hundred kina (about USD$250 then, USD$150 now) each way to hire the health-centre ambulance to take her to the hospital in Buka, a several-hour ride, where she could have the services of an exceptionally good, young Bougainvillean woman obstetrician. From Buin, farther away in the no-go area, the ambulance cost was about the equivalent of five hundred American dollars one way to the hospital. Financial and geographic barriers conspired to cause many delivering women to die.

Hearing about our visit, a local landowner brought us a letter to take back to the National Department of Health in Port Moresby. The woman owned most of the land in Arawa; land inheritance was matrilineal. "My letter threatens to close the Arawa Health Centre if the practice of charging delivering women for the ambulance ride for emergency obstetric care in Buka town isn't stopped. No one can afford five hundred dollars for a one-way ambulance ride, and I'm tired of hearing about these poor pregnant women left to die in Arawa or Buin."

With this degree of challenge, it wasn't surprising that Bougainville was home to several "hot spot" districts — areas where supervised delivery, immunization coverage, or malaria went largely unaddressed. We talked with the doctors in the health centre at Arawa.

"Money from the Global Fund has helped distribute bed nets throughout the country, and deaths from malaria have decreased," we were told. "But the forms we're supposed to use in the antenatal register for prevention of mother to child transmission [PMTCT] for HIV are just a joke. We have no nevirapine available to prevent HIV transmission to the baby. We have no rapid plasma reagin kits to test pregnant women for syphilis. We do have penicillin available to treat that but don't know whom to treat. Keeping mothers from developing advanced syphilis would help prolong their lives. Penicillin would save the lives of their newborns. When our visitors from the national program came last week, they had a helpful piece of advice. They told us to lock up the PMTCT register to protect the privacy of HIV patients. Surely, drugs to treat them and their children would also be important?"

Jens interjected, "Papua New Guinea is terribly challenged with respect to the availability of even simple medicines. You had a corrupt system to procure drugs that flourished under the former permanent secretary of health. Even though the head of the drugs program has been sacked on the basis of embezzlement charges, he's back in office. The PS was also fired, and now he's challenged the decision in the courts. The new PS is only acting and his salary hasn't been regularized. The donors have fought to put an independent expatriate into the system for providing essential drugs, but these efforts have been sabotaged by the bureaucrats who are angry about losing their lucrative business."

We had seen up-country how the stock-outs of basic iron and folic acid to treat the anemia so common in pregnant women had led to preventable deaths in women with even a slight bleed during labour and delivery. Some of the contraceptives in the country contained less than the minimum amount of hormones, bought from unregulated manufacturers without UN approval and leading to contraceptive failure, unwanted pregnancies, illegal abortion, and the deaths of those women who resorted to them. It was no wonder that the death rates of pregnant women in PNG had doubled in the past ten years.

An Australian-funded Papua New Guinean nurse working to help strengthen the health system echoed what we had already discovered. "The anti-retroviral drugs I was given as post-exposure prophylaxis in case of rape, which is too bloody common here, had already expired by the time I was given them. So had the rapid diagnostic test kits for malaria that came one year, paid for by the Global Fund, which had suffered from delays in distribution. Though useful for a short time before they expired, many were wasted. We have no power for microscopes, nor enough lab personnel to read slides to diagnose malaria through blood parasite screening. So these simple rapid tests, which can diagnose two types of malaria in minutes with just a drop of blood on a test strip without a microscope, are essential in rural areas but sadly aren't widely available. Malaria and HIV in pregnancy are major causes of maternal deaths."

After our meeting, we made the same strenuous journey back to Buka. If we were so uncomfortable, how did the more fortunate pregnant women who could scramble to collect hundreds of dollars for the ambulance ride possibly manage lying in labour as they bounced over these impossible roads? Our first stop when we arrived was the UN office.

In the UN's new age of "Delivering as One," the United Nations in Buka delightfully "delivered" the United Nations Development Program, UNICEF, and the World Health Organization, all under the same roof in a single-storey building on the main street. Three different patterns of floral linoleum covered the plywood flooring. Jens and I sat around the conference table with the health team from Bougainville.

One colleague complained, "Every year we're required to write 'annual activity plans.' This is just an empty, meaningless ritual. A new requirement was recently added that the governor had to sign an executive summary introduction to the plan. The Autonomous Region of Bougainville doesn't have a governor, so we couldn't fill this requirement. We had a president, Joe Kabui, who died this year when he couldn't afford medications for his own heart disease."

Bougainville was eligible to receive money from the government of PNG's HSIP (Health Sector Improvement Plan), but it had no governor, even though it had a plan. As of May 2008, no money from the HSIP has been advanced to Bougainville. Had it not been for limited funds from its own government, and from the UN agencies in Bougainville, the health system would have collapsed. In June 2019 the people of Bougainville will vote on independence from PNG, but this will require the reopening of the Panguna Mine, and conflicts persist over who would run that mine. In 2017 the President of Bougainville said the autonomous region would take legal action over the Papua New Guinea government's failure to meet its constitutional commitments on financing.[40]

We replied that in some ways they were better off than some of the other provinces, which still believed they could access HSIP money to allow staff to go for outreach patrols and supervision. But the HSIP was so hamstrung by bureaucracy that little could be used. More money was allocated to the national level of the health system (which didn't implement and had more money than they could spend), but service delivery levels (districts and health centres) were allowed less than half of what they applied for to undertake activities.

Insecurity and weak governance conspire terribly against development progress, even when there is money and goodwill. We left the airport, ducking as a shot rang out, wounding a judge in front of us who had made an unpopular decision. Upon our arrival in our hotel, slightly shaken, a television news report greeted us. The chief pediatrician at Port Moresby General Hospital, Dr. David Mokela, explained, "Two women in PNG die every day and sixty more suffer from pregnancy-related complications because of the tremendous obstacles of lack of roads, deepening poverty, lack of trained health workers, and the closure of many aid posts in rural areas."

I hoped that dedicated health workers like Dr. Mokela could push a government to use its own resources and the generous foreign aid it receives at the bottom where it was most needed. We had certainly failed.

6

I Am Tired of Seeing HIV as the Price of Wealth:

Tanzania and Papua New Guinea

Tanzania, 2002

In the antenatal clinic of a small district hospital in Tanzania, about sixty women, at least half of them appearing to be teenagers, sat patiently, crowded close together, on low wooden benches. I had seen varying versions of this weary patient group of women in countless countries in Sub-Saharan Africa, differentiated by clothing and tribal face markings. There were about forty kids with their mothers, the little ones in satchels on their mothers' backs, and the toddlers sitting quietly at knee level beside their mothers. At least ten of the mothers were breastfeeding. One tired midwife was trying to screen the women, glancing up every few minutes with a grim, discouraged smile as even more women came into the waiting area, replacing the ones she had already seen and making the line seem interminable. Around the corner was another waiting area, but this one was spacious. It had been recently painted and was bright and cheerful. Three midwives attended those patients. There were seven women waiting for their HIV test results. A brand-new CD4 cell count machine hummed busily in the lab adjacent to the clinic.

I tucked my head in to see Lily, the midwife who was screening the prenatals. I had brought her a cup of tea in a slightly chipped white mug. "I won't keep you. I know you're busy."

"Busy? Look around the corner. Those midwives make three times as much as I do. They were hired with AIDS money. No one can be hired on the regular service because of the freeze, but the donors made a special arrangement for AIDS. Of course, midwives left the routine work to go and work in HIV. Three times more money! We have even less staff than before."[1]

Lily's voice dropped; it was full of bitterness. She switched to Swahili and tried to smile as she turned back to her patient, who was coming for her first visit, at about seven months. "When you come back here to deliver, you'll have to bring supplies. Bring Jik bleach, gloves, sutures, a razor blade. You'll also need a pad to cover you after you deliver, and a rubber sheet for the bed. For pain you can bring acetaminophen."

She turned to me again as I was leaving her room. "Look at this woman. This is Sarah. She's poor, and her husband has lost his job. The number of poor people is increasing. They have to pay to register. Care for pregnant women is supposed to be free, but we have no supplies. And only a quarter of the facilities in the country even have water.[2] It isn't surprising that women deliver at home."

I returned to the clinic two months later. I had come to design support to reduce HIV — a large World Bank grant had been given to all sectors, with health as the lead ministry. This was a multi-sectoral AIDS support program: money was to be allotted to several government ministries, including health, education, and women and children's affairs. Large grants were also provided to NGOs and civil society groups for grassroots supports for prevention, care, and treatment, and to impact mitigation such as help for orphans and vulnerable groups.

When Lily saw me, she asked, "Remember that woman Sarah? I was screening her when we spoke last. I remember her. She stands out in my mind. She was so bright and well spoken. Do you know what happened to that woman? She died. She tried to deliver at home and ran into trouble. She started to bleed. It took too long for her to get money for an ambulance, and she couldn't get the money to pay for a C-section. She died just after she got here. I was on the OB floor last week when they brought her in."

Lily shook her head in sorrow and frustration, her lips fixed in a furious straight line, her brow deeply furrowed. I took both of Lily's hands and clasped them in my own. I imagined that those warm hands were sharing strength. I thanked her for her time and returned by Jeep to Dar es Salaam.

Back in Dar, I spoke with Maggie Bangser, who headed the Women's Dignity Project, an NGO that addressed maternal health and the prevention and treatment of obstetric fistula. I said to her, "I thought there were supposed to be exemptions for maternal health. It's supposed to be free. Why are women being charged for the basic supplies to give birth?"

Maggie quoted the Demographic and Health Survey (DHS), which showed the various barriers women faced and the problem of maternal exemptions (free care that facilities are supposed to provide, but they don't often get reimbursed so they stop providing the care).

We also discussed the hiring freeze on health workers.[3] This had been required to reduce the money paid for salaries so that Tanzania could pay off its debts. There had been cuts in the budget for operating costs. But global health initiatives had brought in huge amounts of money for HIV/AIDS, and the government had been given permission for special hiring to deal with the new needs of HIV.[4] This had led the treasury to reduce money for other health sector priorities.[5]

Maggie's group had hired Paul Smithson to analyze the problems more deeply.[6] Women's Dignity had already brought Davidson Gwatkin (from 2000–3, he was the World Bank's principal health and poverty specialist) to Tanzania to discuss inequities in maternal health. He had reviewed the DHS, which showed that one woman died every hour in Tanzania giving birth. The DHS had reported that the majority of women had at least one prenatal visit, but less than half could afford to deliver in a health facility. And poor women were seven times more likely to deliver at home than richer women. Clearly, there were major barriers that poor women faced.

The Public Expenditure Review, which analyzed where government and donor money actually went, had discovered that more than a third of the money in the health sector had come from donors, and that was going up. It had been one quarter. But a lot of that money was earmarked for HIV. Nearly one-third of all the donor money coming in to Tanzania was for HIV/AIDS.[7]

This meant that Tanzania had to cut back on the money spent on medical supplies, forcing patients to bring their own supplies. It hadn't been possible to get enough money to poor districts to enable them to hire more staff, even though the country had district allocation grants that allowed additional money for poor districts as one effort to improve equity. So there were inequalities in the availability of health workers. Poor areas couldn't compete. Health had received less government money from the treasury, and the health sector was penalized because so much money was coming in for HIV, mostly for care and treatment with expensive anti-retroviral drugs.[8]

This created a dilemma. Reducing HIV decreased the deaths of pregnant women related to HIV, but the balance wasn't right. In 2006 the deaths of pregnant women appeared to be going up, and fewer women were having safe deliveries attended by a midwife. Tanzania still had high rates of teenage pregnancy, which made those teens at higher risk. A stronger condom promotion strategy would help prevent AIDS as well as high-risk pregnancy.

I spoke to my colleague, Dr. Njau, at the Ministry of Health, who furrowed his brow and frowned. "Tanzania has high rates of maternal deaths, and women have a one-in-twenty-three risk of dying in labour.[9] In part, we have so little money. We spend just over seven dollars per person a year on health. The minimum required is over thirty dollars."[10]

I replied, "Two thirds of the money you receive for HIV goes for treatment, which is costly. The funds you receive keep going up, but less than 15 percent is for prevention, and more of this goes to abstain-and-be-faithful messages than for condom use."[11]

I left Dr. Njau's office and headed to one of the Ministry of Health's portable buildings, which housed small offices, including my own. I unlocked the door to my cubicle and tossed my briefcase onto the desk. Why should health workers in HIV make so much more money so that there were even fewer midwives to deliver babies safely? I was here to help program money for reducing HIV. How could we use this money to strengthen health systems more broadly to benefit the people of Tanzania?

Grabbing a pen and a pad of foolscap paper, I jotted some quick notes before I started to work at the computer, moving outside my portable to sit in the sun. A peacock strolled by, ignoring me completely. A few colleagues from the Ministry of Health walked by, engaged in Swahili conversation, interrupting themselves to ask in cheerful English, "Are you all right? Do you have malaria? You are sitting in the sun. We only do that when we are sick."

I nodded that I was okay. Two hours had passed since I had spoken with Dr. Njau. Somewhere in Tanzania two women had died in labour. Maybe I was sick — at heart. The sun would do little to ease that sickness.

———

In 2008 the U.S. government spent 60 percent of its funding for global health on HIV/AIDS.[12] That year only 27 percent of U.S. aid for global health was earmarked for maternal and child health. In 2010, 7.6 million children under five died in developing countries, while twelve thousand fewer children perished daily in 2010 than in 1990.[13] Four hundred thousand mothers die annually, many leaving orphaned infants also at risk of dying, while 1.8 million people die from AIDS annually.[14] For 2012, from U.S. government support to their global commitments, $6 billion went to HIV (mostly treatment), $846 million to maternal and child health, and $625 million to family planning.[15] Per foreign assistance, in 2017 the U.S. spent $3.77 billion on HIV/AIDS and $893.6 million on maternal and child health.

According to the World Health Report 2005, between 1990–92 and 2000–2, the share of external official flows (funding from all donors for health) that was allocated for maternal and reproductive health increased from 30 percent to 39 percent, representing a doubling, from US$1 to $2 billion per year.[16] But this primarily reflected an increase in funding for HIV/AIDS. Monies for family planning and maternal health from many key donors such as the United States decreased in relative and absolute terms in the same period.[17]

Authors such as Jeremy Shiffman (associate professor of public administration, Syracuse University) have emphasized that maternal health advocates could make a better case for mobilizing resources.[18] Roger England in the British Medical Journal in 2007 argued we are spending too much on HIV and not on other causes of illness and deaths, including mother-and-child health.[19]

There have been efforts to improve synergy such as strengthening health systems to better deliver maternal health as well as support for HIV/AIDS, for example, with health systems support from the Global Fund.

But in every country I have worked in, the balance leans much more heavily toward HIV and has directed health workers away from maternal health toward HIV efforts. And within the HIV efforts, more funding has gone to costly treatment instead of prevention, which could also reduce high-risk adolescent pregnancies.

PAPUA NEW GUINEA, 2008

The Air Niugini flight from Brisbane, Australia, to Port Moresby, Papua New Guinea, had been downgraded to a smaller plane. All eighteen seats were occupied. Five of us were women. In addition to two Papua New Guinean flight attendants, there were three expatriate women, including me, on the plane.

I chatted with my seatmate, an Australian in shorts and sandals who was managing the construction of housing in mine sites throughout PNG. I asked if he knew about HIV in the country. Did he know that HIV prevalence was increasing and was now a generalized epidemic? Did he know that almost 1.5 percent of all adults were HIV positive?

Bart didn't know but wasn't concerned. "No worries, mate. I don't sleep around."

Two weeks later I was in Lae, Morobe, a gold-mining area. Two slightly drunk Australian men in shorts, T-shirts, and waterproof sandals, reminiscent of the one I had met on the plane, had driven up to the bar in a pickup truck. They went into the bar. Five minutes later they came out with six very drunk Papua New Guinean women who appeared to be in their late teens. The men grabbed the giggling women and threw them, squealing like pigs, into the back of the pickup. The women wore tight jeans and worn flip-flop sandals. Poorly applied lipstick stained their cigarettes. For a night's work, expatriate customers paid more than locals; these women could expect the price of a bottle of cheap wine.

These dynamics have had terrible consequences: Papua New Guinea is the leading country for HIV in the South Pacific. The sudden injection of money (and men) for resource exploitation has been a huge social challenge to an impoverished culture where many are still trading yams. Access to both treatment and prevention is improving but still challenged, and there has been difficulty reaching those most at risk as well as analyzing funds spent on HIV activities in a rigorous way so that priority areas can receive the most resources. Scandals of money mismanagement plague the National HIV/AIDS Secretariat.

But there were many signs of hope, of money coming in where it was needed. Topa was with Save the Children Fund in PNG and informed me over dinner one evening, "We failed the USAID 'ABC' audit! We were working with high-risk groups, men who have sex with men or sex workers. But USAID said too much of our project was 'C' or condom distribution, not enough 'A' (abstain) or 'B' (be faithful) for the Bush administration. Luckily, the Australian and New Zealand governments have a more pragmatic approach. They have re-funded us."

The next week I was back in Port Moresby and talking with Kel, who worked for the Asian Development Bank. He told me, "We have six 'rural development enclaves' [such as oil, and mining], which have developed primary health care services, including HIV prevention and treatment, around their economic ventures. This public/private partnership is showing huge successes. It's still tough. There have been a lot of delays and red tape. This has slowed our work with building rehabilitation, as well as with training and the distribution of medicines. But overall we're making progress. We had an excellent evaluation and will be expanding the model to other enclave areas and strengthening other activities beyond HIV such as malaria and TB control.

"We know that urban areas are getting worse and that the enclaves have to take the lead. In some urban clinics for sexually transmitted infection, nearly 15 percent of the patients are HIV positive, a rate which has tripled from 2002. And we want to do more with pregnant women. Three percent of pregnant women in two provinces are HIV positive. We're also trying to work with the Catholic Church. In some of the Catholic dioceses a fifth of the people attending for voluntary counselling and testing are positive."[20]

Kel also had some interesting, less technical stories. The context of sexuality in PNG had some unusual features. In most of the festivals, tattooed, feathered, painted, and grass-skirted women of all ages danced bare-breasted. Western cultures' preoccupation with breasts and genitals didn't apply here. Beauty in the eye of the beholder had a different meaning.

Sara was a friend of Kel's. One Saturday night she was swimming with Edai, a missionary friend of hers from the Mission Aviation Fellowship in Papua. Sara told me a story that Edai had shared at one of their missionary meetings. A guy stood up and said that when he was visiting a mission in the Highlands he was horrified to see a bunch of Papuan men — Dani or Ikar (two PNG tribes in that area) — reading a girlie magazine. They were very animated, these men who were traditionally dressed wearing only boars' tusks in their noses and *koteka* (penis gourds/sheaths).

The American missionary rushed over to do something — an intervention. He discouraged them from these magazines, which objectified women. But he found out that what they were discussing was the naked woman's teeth. They were trying to work out whether she had an even or uneven number (for Ikari or Dani, only even numbers are good, which means educators have to use even numbers in teaching materials). Nudity was normal. It was the number of teeth that could be upsetting.

***

HIV has a great deal of visibility. Since PNG has the highest HIV rates in the South Pacific, there is an increase in funding to try to reduce infection. But there have been difficulties due to thinking in "silos." A large grant from the Global Fund (which works to reduce HIV, tuberculosis, and malaria) could have been structured to help strengthen prenatal care, linked with the provision of anti-malarial drugs. A project from Australia and New Zealand built free-standing STD clinics, which were underutilized, set off at a distance behind walls from the prenatal ward, while crowded antenatal clinics lacked staff or supplies to test for syphilis, a sexually transmitted infection. The Global Fund grant didn't address STDs, though these increase the likelihood of HIV transmission. Grant requests are developed by national governments such as PNG's, with external technical assistance. So we are all responsible if we have created a fragmented system full of gaps and duplications. There are many missed opportunities to strengthen a health system and improve care for pregnant women by integrating antenatal care with malaria prevention and detection of syphilis and HIV.

Projects such as the Asian Development Bank's Rural Enclaves Project are planning to build on the entry point of HIV prevention. The intention is to see if prenatal care and trained midwives can also be supported to help the communities around mines and plantations. But this is a harder sell for some companies. Keeping their workers from getting HIV makes economic sense; saving the community women's lives from dying in labour needs a stronger level of corporate social responsibility. The project was deemed to be largely successful: the final evaluation deemed the project to be relevant, effective, sustainable, and to have had impact on HIV prevention and skilled birth attendance, but to have had problems with efficiency, such as lower social marketing of condoms than expected.[21]

———————

Missionaries often had to take on unusual roles in these countries. Just as Father Brendan in Zimbabwe was an advocate for family planning and safe sex, so, too, was Father Paul, whom I met in Papua New Guinea distributing condoms in his diocese to fight against AIDS. On a visit to Karema in Gulf Province, I was out for a stroll with Mark, an Australian colleague. Our steps took us back along the soccer field, past the market with twenty or so women under umbrellas selling betel nuts, lychees, bananas, slices of watermelon, coconuts, boiled eggs, smoked fish, yarn in bright colours, packets of razor blades, and blocks of soap, all laid out on squares of cloth. Ahead of us we saw a large house painted yellow, blue, green, red, and black, with strange Papua New Guinean designs — masked, costumed dancers and large bright birds. Curious, we walked over, and just beside the house we saw a church with a roof and no walls but instead an open grillwork of wrought iron in designs of flowers, sunrays, and birds. At the entrance of the church was a giant clamshell broader than the length of my arm, which held holy water to bless oneself.

Inside, a Mass had just started. Six priests were preparing Communion at the altar, beside which two rectangular stained glass windows glowed with wild colours. The congregation was composed of a handful of Papua

New Guineans in informal clothes. In two rows toward the back were about ten nuns wearing folds of white, edged with three blue stripes on the left-hand border, draped over their heads and flowing down their bodies. I was reminded of Mother Teresa, and indeed they belonged to the Missionaries of Charity order.

It had been years since I had been to Mass. I had to go in; it was such a welcoming scene with wonderful singing. My Anglican colleague stayed on the porch, looking out over the water and mist-shrouded hills, palm trees, and children playing on the shore, while I slipped inside and knelt at the nearest pew. It felt so good to be there, wafted along by the comforting ritual. My voice joined the others in song and prayer. The church was so open, the breeze blowing through, the feeling of peace so tangible; I flowed through Communion.

After the Mass, Mark and I chatted with the senior priest, who was from Alsace-Lorraine and who had been in PNG since 1963. He described the work of the diocese with the youth, running hospitals and schools. Then he pointed across the courtyard to Father Paul, "the African priest," who was the HIV/AIDS coordinator. Father Paul worked in a neighbouring district that we wouldn't be able to visit since the airstrip was closed, so we seized the opportunity to ask him about his work.

The African priest was tall and slim, and exuded quiet grace. He smiled with delight to learn I had been to his birthplace, a district in Uganda. Father Paul described his work passionately. "I came here as a missionary to PNG because I've seen the devastation that AIDS can bring to a country, to families, and to villages, and I needed to warn my parishioners here. I've established a voluntary counselling and testing centre but have nothing to offer those who test positive. There are no anti-retroviral drugs, which cost only a few dollars, not even to prevent the pregnant women from passing on the infection to their babies. And there is a deep background of violence against women here that is fuelling the epidemic. The women in my parish face rapes and beatings, and I have had to personally intervene against men abusing their wives." Then, suddenly, he became more enthusiastic. "The young people are teaching each other about HIV in song and drama."

Father Paul worried about the AIDS orphans he was trying to care for with limited resources. To help pay the expenses for his centre, he had built a fee-charging guest house on the second floor for visitors to his district because, of course, the initial funding had dried up when the original project had ended. Somehow the massive amounts of money for HIV coming into PNG weren't getting to this district. Promised visits from the national HIV coordinators hadn't yet materialized, and no one in his district could afford to travel to the capital for treatment.

HIV treatment required technical backstopping such as CD4 cell count machines; small rural health facilities with no electricity would never be able to offer HIV treatment. Bureaucratic bottlenecks meant that only specially trained counsellors could offer pregnant women voluntary counselling and testing. Poor areas had fewer staff and couldn't afford to send any of those people away for training, since that would have left them even more underserviced. The skew that was seen in treating HIV paralleled the distortion in other aspects of health such as maternal care. Antenatal care, midwives at delivery, and emergency obstetric care were easier to access if a woman was urban, educated, and wealthy. So it was very difficult to get care for a woman in a poor rural area.

Father Paul's eyes shone brightly as he recounted the story of one woman being treated in Port Moresby who had been nearing death but was now strong. He had found the money for her travel, but her husband had died because Father Paul could only come up with money for one of them. I was reminded of women with too many children who allowed the youngest to die of malnutrition, so they would be able to care for the rest. I was reminded how very tough the choices could be in development and health care.

Self-taught as a health worker, Father Paul did rapid HIV tests and voluntary counselling and testing and managed home-based care. I asked him about condoms. Although the Vatican and his bishop were reluctant to allow their use even for disease prevention, Father Paul ensured they were distributed in his diocese. He knew that condoms kept parents alive to take care of their children. Father Paul was doing so much, with so few resources, that we promised we would follow up in the capital for him, particularly since there had been no anti-retroviral drugs available in the provincial hospital, either.

Mark and I then glanced at each other but stayed silent. We felt humbled by Father Paul's commitment. The priest explained that vocations were increasing in Africa, and more clerics like himself were coming out to countries such as PNG as missionaries.

Just as many of the HIV experts in the U.N. agencies in Papua New Guinea were from Africa — Zambia, Ghana, Uganda, Tanzania — there was a groundswell of response from Sub-Saharan Africa, which has the highest HIV rates in the world, to help other countries at an earlier stage of the epidemic. It was so hopeful to see these shining lights in the world: the woman doctor organizing prevention of parent-to-child transmission services was from Zambia; several experts at WHO and UNICEF were from Tanzania, working to help HIV orphans; and one doctor from Ghana, who knew Jens well, was helping the Papua New Guineans to manage their Global Fund grant. I had met experts from countries such as Botswana working in the Caribbean, the second worst hit HIV region after Sub-Saharan Africa. This type of south-south collaboration, with people from developing countries sharing their expertise with one another, was a solid and practical way to facilitate the learning curve and move countries forward.

To thank Father Paul for his commitment and dedication, I went the next morning early to give a small offering for his work and found, at 6:45 a.m., a Mass again being held. So for the second time I shared in Communion and felt strengthened. My journey with the Roman Catholic Church has been a strange dance. When the Vatican sided with Islamic fundamentalists to block reproductive rights for women at the Cairo Conference on Population and Development in 1994 (I had written the background paper for the Canadian delegation, showcasing CIDA's support to Bangladesh), I moved away from the church, weary of the battle fatigue when I was fighting for contraception. But on many occasions when I have been exhausted with the slow pace of change and the challenges of fighting systems based on money, the church has been a safe refuge upholding the rights and dignity of the poor.

After Mass I stood quietly with tall, graceful Father Paul as serene nuns from the Missionaries of Charity filed out and nodded at him respectfully. A few Papua New Guineans also greeted him, some placing a hand on his arm or nodding silently as they passed. I asked Father Paul how he kept from being discouraged.

He was slow to answer. Still smiling as the parishioners passed him, he finally answered calmly, "My life of prayer. I wouldn't have become a priest if I didn't believe. I've seen what HIV did to my own country. I also saw that even a poor country like Uganda could dramatically reduce HIV. In Uganda the churches helped to advocate for young people to delay having sex, and for greater fidelity. And that worked. The health sector and NGOs worked to make condoms more available. These were complementary efforts. The reduction in high-risk adolescent pregnancies in Uganda helped to save women's lives, and this was a spin-off of the HIV prevention effort. We can do the same here in PNG.

"You have to have a holistic approach. Women are vulnerable here, even though they have such great strength. They can't refuse sex with their husbands. Women become weakened from frequent childbearing, and the death rates of pregnant women are going up as the health system deteriorates and poverty worsens. Even though the public health system is trying to emphasize reducing HIV and the deaths of pregnant women, both problems are getting worse."

Many of my friends in PNG admitted frankly that their motivation was financial. PNG was a hardship post, especially for women because of the risk of rape and HIV, so there were bonuses and career fast-tracking to reward working in the country. But Father Paul had no such rewards. He supported many AIDS orphans with his own money and was often in conflict with his own church supervisors because of his liberal attitudes. But he tirelessly fought on. "We did it in Uganda," he told me again. "And we can do it in PNG. We should never forget the power of hope."

7

WHERE ARE OUR LEADERS?
WHY HAVE THEY FORGOTTEN US?

MALAWI, PAPUA NEW GUINEA, GHANA,
AND A GLOBAL REFLECTION

MALAWI, 1990

I returned from my journeys in Africa, Asia, and the South Pacific more conscious of both the vulnerability and the resilience of women in poor countries. But they were at the mercy of the political leadership in their nations, leaders who could ensure money was directed to mother-and-child health or embezzle it for their own purposes. So few women were in positions of leadership. Women were leaders in their communities informally — wise traditional birth attendants, supports to one another with family stresses — but didn't have real political power or the ability to command resources. Would women with that kind of leverage make a difference in the priorities of poor countries?

In 1990, beside a pool in a well-appointed hotel in Lilongwe, Malawi, I met a clean-shaven man named Paul and introduced myself, explaining that I, a newcomer to Malawi, was here to plan district primary health care — mother-and-child health, HIV/AIDS prevention and treatment, clean water and sanitation — and to assess the training of medical assistants in orthopedic surgery.

Speaking with a careful upper-class British accent, he looked up from the pocket mystery book he was reading and told me there was a very ugly underbelly to every story I would hear. "People disappear in the night, never to be seen again. They're watched and then killed violently by the secret service." He explained that the trail moved up from the secret police all the way to the highly placed officials I'd already started meeting in the Ministry of Health. Some had OBE (Order of the British Empire) after their names, and some were living as royalty in the presidential palace. This was life under Hastings Kamuzu Banda, the "Life President" of Malawi.

But the country was actually run by his official consort, Mama Kadzamira, the architect of Banda's career and the real power behind the throne. Paul gave me his perspective. "Banda is carefully surrounded by handlers who make sure he sees only what's permissible and is kept sheltered from the grim realities of the country. The English secretary who left her husband for him has conveniently died in poverty. Mama Kadzamira runs the show now. If she and her cronies bring him to see a hospital, they only show him one ward, paint it up nicely, and show only the healthiest patients. I doubt he even knows there's an HIV epidemic."

Paul wore a conservative, royal blue bathing suit and was handsome in a James Bond kind of way, with just the suggestion of a cleft chin, a trace of a five o'clock shadow, piercing blue-green eyes, and a nicely tanned, well-muscled torso. "Although the origins of the name Malawi remain unclear, the name is said to mean the "glitter of the sun rising across the lake" — Lake Malawi, which shares borders with Mozambique, Malawi, and Tanzania, and lies in the Great African Rift Valley. It is the third-largest lake in Africa and the ninth largest in the world."

The next day I left Lilongwe and its luxury hotels and arrived at a small camp overlooking the lake where I was to stay. I took my gin and tonic sundowner alone and watched hippos emerge from the water. I had unpacked my few well-chosen clothes (it was illegal for women to wear trousers; skirts had to go below the knee). Night was full of the rustling sounds of lizards skittering along the walls, as well as the humming of mosquitoes hitting the slightly tattered netting over my bed.

In the morning, two uniformed health department midwives from the local health office collected me in a Jeep, and we spent the day visiting health centres and a small hospital. I was saddened by the crowded wards, the women who had developed obstetric fistula from obstructed births, the wasted, malnourished kids, and the thin, coughing HIV and TB patients.

Soon after, I began to catch glimpses of the ugly underbelly Paul had mentioned. I was visiting Pia, a Danish doctor who lived down the road from my hippo camp. Having worked with Jens, it felt comfortable to be around someone who kept switching into Danish, momentarily forgetting I was English-speaking.

Pia's cook, Mr. Bangula, asked for a medical excuse for his wife to release her from being drafted as one of the group of women who accompanied Banda and his entourage as "official praise singers." Mr. Bangula was distressed. "These women wear Banda's face on their kanga cloth dresses, and sing and dance ecstatically as the Supreme Ruler tours his kingdom. But the women who are drafted for this role have to sleep with anyone in the official party. No, I don't want my wife to leave me for this role, though the president's office said I should be proud."

Pia and I wrote the letter, explaining fictitiously that Mr. Bangula's wife couldn't be considered because her asthma would be exacerbated by long hours of dancing and singing, and her diabetes required more regular meals than she would have while travelling.

As we were talking, there was a peremptory knock at the door. Brown-uniformed members of the youth wing of the ruling party were goose-stepping from house to house to collect money. Pia explained with a nervous smile, "Failure to donate leads to later visits, beatings, and thefts, so both Africans and expatriates manage to come up with the contributions we hope will be sufficient."

Days later, on July 6, 1990, I was once again visiting Pia for homemade cinnamon rolls and to celebrate the glorious Day of Independence, recalling the martyrs who had lost their lives in the fight against the British colonial rulers in 1964. Pia handed me a platter of steaming, buttery rolls and advised, "Expats have to stay home today because there may be incidents."

Pia had several friends over, and they were celebrating the day watching *Out of Africa* on video, somewhat incongruous given the colonial view of history in the movie that juxtaposed with the African celebration of independence from British rule, albeit in Kenya instead of Malawi.

The fact was that very few "martyrs" died in the relatively peaceful hand-over in Malawi from colonial rule. The vehemently anti-British rhetoric came from the despotic Banda. Officially born in 1906, he took the name Hastings after being baptized into the Church of Scotland. In his late teens he walked from Malawi (then called Nyasaland) to Zimbabwe (then called Rhodesia), then on to South Africa. He worked in the mines until he met a Methodist benefactor who paid for his American schooling from 1925 to 1928. After that he went to premedical and then medical studies in the United States, supported by various patrons, including heirs to the empires of Eastman Kodak and Pepsodent. Banda later trained in Scotland and worked as a doctor in England. Eventually, he returned to Malawi in 1958, after a brief scandal involving his secretary, who left her husband for him. Banda was imprisoned in 1959 when Rhodesian troops invaded the increasingly aggressive Nyasaland. He continued to fight for independence and for his own autocratic power, and he was rewarded in 1971 by being declared President for Life.[1]

Banda affected a slightly pompous and frivolous air, with his three-piece suits and matching kerchiefs and fly whisk, and he endeavoured to maintain an image as benevolent and eccentric or simply vain — certainly not evil. He was rumoured to be increasingly senile. He might not have been aware of the death squads run by his official hostess, Mama Kadzamira, or of the vast wealth she was accumulating. Every building had to have his official photograph. All media, including *Time* and *Newsweek*, were censored. There were strict dress codes for women.

The following day Pia and I visited local communities that were installing running water and sanitation in their villages and learning how to conduct safer deliveries. We visited the health facilities and checked the skills of the hard-working, underpaid health workers. I spent one morning in the mud hut of a traditional birth attendant, seeing how carefully she delivered the women who came to her, how well kept her home was, how clean. We later visited one small community and were ushered onto grass mats and chairs under a tree to listen to the local dance troupe sing AIDS prevention songs being used for health education. HIV/AIDS was a major cause of maternal deaths, as was malaria.

In the afternoon, Pia left for home to have dinner with her husband and two lovely daughters. I changed my clothes and shifted emotional gears. I was travelling now with Dr. Ed Blair, an orthopedic surgeon on a Canadian-funded project, up a long, curving, tree-lined drive past uniformed guards to the presidential palace for tea. Across from us was a graceful, glittering sweep of blue and green on the ceremonial lawns, a haughty arabesque as the tame peacocks reminded us that we, too, were on display.

Watchful. Unlucky. Vain. Violent. Evil.

Words used to represent these peacocks in myth and legend. Words that were seeping into my mind. There was a dangerous undertone in every situation. I felt off balance, wary.

Three of us were eating pancakes, Canadian maple syrup, crustless cucumber sandwiches, and tea. Dr. Blair was a frequent visitor to the palace. He had ignored me when I tried to tell him about some of the more nefarious undertakings of his good friends, the leaders of Malawi. "She uses her power well," Dr. Blair said. "You women's libbers complain there aren't enough women in politics and then you complain again when things don't progress fast enough for you. Make up your frigging minds."

Mama Kadzamira was, after all, the patron of Dr. Blair's Rotary-funded project that I was evaluating, and our hostess. We had recommended that the medical assistants trained to do orthopedic surgery also be taught to perform Caesarean sections. In a small hospital they might be the only staff that could operate to save a woman's life from obstructed labour.

Several tall white-jacketed waiters stood ready to serve. I wore an inexpensive but showy satin cocktail dress, a white-and-hot-pink tropical print that met the regulations and came to just above mid-calf. Mama Kadzamira offered us more tea. In a regal voice, with modest undertones, she explained, "I was a nurse working in the United Kingdom when I met him, a doctor. He is now not well and is only brought out for official tours."

I tried not to think of the role of Banda and Mama Kadzamira in the disappearances and death squads. We discussed some concerns. A Canadian charity had donated some used clothing for Mozambican refugees living in Malawi. Instead the clothes were sold at the request of Mama Kadzamira, the proceeds used to buy two dialysis machines and the reagent chemicals used in the infusions. These were kept for a lucky few affluent patients, wealthy people who could afford dialysis, or senior state visitors with renal failure who might need medical care. Mama

Kadzamira assured me this was her wise decision, a good cause, too, as good as that of the refugees. I asked about other needs, including high rates of malnutrition and under-equipped health centres, attempting to keep my voice as carefully modulated and level as her own. She was elegantly and expensively dressed and carried her plumpness with grace. Nodding and with her eyes partially closed, she looked like a huge bullfrog sunning herself on a lily pad.

"My dear young woman, you cannot possibly understand. This is just your first visit here? I assure you that what little malnutrition exists is 'cultural.' It is due to ignorance, as are the deaths of young children from diarrhea, pneumonia, and measles. I agree it really is a pity. The mothers simply do not know how to look after their little ones. And they are like animals. They just squat down and deliver their babies at home. It is a shame, really. We do what we can. I, myself, have several charities."

I sensed she expected us to be grateful and beholden to her that she had granted us this audience. She was so insulated and had cloaked herself with charitable concerns like the Canadian-funded project, hence CIDA's suggestion I might need a dress in case I was invited to the palace. Mama Kadzamira was also the patron of another Rotary-assisted project — Malawi Against Polio — besides the one training medical assistants.

The Rotary Club in Canada had warned me about Dr. Blair. "He hates women doctors. He hates McMaster Medical School. And he hates the New Democratic Party [a social democratic party in Canada]."

When I arrived and Dr. Blair met me off the plane, I had stretched out my right hand to greet him. "Hi, I'm your worst nightmare. A New Democrat, trained at McMaster, and I'm here to evaluate your project."

Dr. Ed Blair had left Canada when the NDP government banned extra billing, which cut into his considerable income as an orthopedic surgeon. Extra billing had been allowed by the Conservative government of the time and had enabled specialists to charge the government as well as their patients for the same service. Yet here Blair was working for a fraction of his former income helping Malawi.

He and I formed an uneasy collaborative working partnership from the start. Conflict between us was inevitable. He had advised me, without irony, that "there is no malnutrition" in Malawi. Blair had spent more time with his friends at the palace than on the pediatric wards. He showed me the orthopedic wards. I agreed he was an excellent trainer of non-doctors to do orthopedic surgery. I showed him the malnourished children dying on the pediatric wards and in the villages with their worried parents. In this area, one in five children would die of hunger before they reached the age of five, or they would succumb to easily treated or prevented illnesses such as diarrhea and measles. By 2015, this had greatly improved: one in sixteen children does not live to their fifth birthday.[2]

Blair and I disagreed about news coverage. The heavily censored newspapers wrote that Banda, the Supreme Ruler, had declared that his official crop inspection tour revealed the best maize crop ever. The paper quoted one visiting ambassador complimenting Malawi for being self-sufficient in food. I argued that this couldn't possibly be true. During our hours of driving between hospitals and health centres, I pointed out the "best maize crop ever" was burned brown in the fields from the lack of rain. That year's crop was lost and the previous year's harvest stores had long been finished. I showed him the many people on the side of the road who were selling food, still with the UN's World Food Programme logos on the containers, obviously on the black market.

We met anxious village women, many of them pregnant and malnourished, whose husbands worked as indentured workers on Banda's vast estates (most assets in the country were somehow under his control and that of his official conglomerate, Press Holdings). The village men weren't allowed to leave these estates until the end of the harvest because they had been "loaned" a bag of maize they needed to pay off. Even though their own children were starving, they weren't able to earn money until the end of the season, by which time some of their children would have died. Nor was this alleged self-sufficiency reflected in the massive food aid given by the World Food Programme. Large tracts of arable land were devoted to vast tobacco plantations owned by Press Holdings, instead of being used to plant food.

The worried villagers were everywhere, but few risked telling us these stories. People were clearly aware that Secret Service informers included our drivers. Well away from our driver, one medical colleague whispered some of his worries about suspected embezzlement of funds from the country's national AIDS control program, headed by one of Mama Kadzamira's friends.

A British doctor told me uncomfortably that he was upset when four of Banda's political enemies were brought to hospital dead on arrival. My British colleague knew that to stay in the country and to continue to provide good medical care to needy people he could neither mention the gunshot wounds on the bodies nor comment when he saw the deaths described in the official press as an unfortunate road traffic accident. This doctor told me this while we sipped sundowners at an elegant cocktail and dinner party. He was dressed in a light tropical suit. The doctor and his athletic, silver-haired wife had been in Malawi for years, carefully screening what they knew, what they saw, what they discussed. He was a surgeon, and there were very few with his level of skill in Malawi. If the brutal truths became too difficult to bear and he had to leave, his absence would deny essential surgical care to the poor.

As we sipped our tea at the presidential palace, Mama Kadzamira continued with a slight sigh, "Ignorance is also fuelling the HIV epidemic. Fourteen percent of our adults have the disease. This is based on estimates from sentinel surveillance of healthy pregnant women and the percentage of donated blood from healthy donors that have to be rejected once found positive. A very good friend of mine is running the national HIV program. We are doing our level best."

We couldn't ignore the HIV rates when, the next day, Dr. Blair and I were in the operating room. Many cases in the theatre supervised by Dr. Blair were HIV positive. Some of these were soldiers, who had higher rates of HIV thanks to long absences from home and frequent access to commercial sex workers, the majority of whom were HIV positive.

As we visited the hospital to assess orthopedic training of clinical officers, one orthopedic assistant proudly introduced us to a soldier whose leg he had saved. "This man is a hero. His leg was blown up and mutilated when he was patrolling trains in Mozambique that were attacked by the

South Africa–backed RENAMO — the Mozambican National Resistance in Portuguese: Resistência Nacional Moçambicana — fighters. But, Dr. Blair, I remembered your rules for how to assess if the limb could be saved. I opposed the doctor on call. But I was right! You taught me well. The leg was viable. I hope he isn't HIV. I nicked myself in the theatre." The orthopedic assistant looked at the forefinger on his left hand and, laughing, licked a small red line running along the finger.

Standing in our greens in the operating room, I was surprised that the doctors and nurses had such a surprisingly casual attitude toward their own accidental injuries such as a nick from a scalpel, which might involve possible infection. It would be too difficult to continue the work if they allowed themselves to worry. Yet the chances of infection were high, and they knew that. I was grateful that I wasn't scrubbed in but was only observing the skill of the trainee medical assistant and the surgeon who was teaching him.

These medical assistants doing orthopedic surgery were saving lives and staying in their small hospitals. They weren't doctors who could leave for more lucrative jobs in other countries. I decided this was a good project and argued with CIDA to continue it. Canada paid one modest salary for an orthopedic surgeon. Many others came from Canada, the United States, and Britain as volunteers to help him teach. There was a terrific multiplier effect with this low-budget project.

I closed my eyes. Did drinking tea at the palace with a woman who ordered opponents to be killed compromise my integrity? I prepared to leave Malawi, carefully folding that fancy dress into my well-worn signature carry-on — the one I always travelled with. I thought to myself, *I've never met dictators before. I've never met people who controlled so many people's lives.* I looked out at the well-paved roads that had many boasting about the success story of Malawi. I saw a thinly disguised, well-run police state where people lived carefully and fearfully.

Only five years later, though, these same people tried to convict Banda and Mama Kadzamira of ordering the assassination of four political opponents in 1983. That time, democracy and the rule of law were unsuccessful.[3]

But by 2001, those dangerous despotic rulers, together with their aide John Tembo, were convicted of fraud and misappropriation of millions of dollars during their eighteen-year reign. Women can gain positions of power as leaders, and when they get there, be just as evil and willing as men to let poor women and children die.

Other successive vice-presidents and presidents had been charged with corruption, and drought and lost crops continue to plague the country. In 2013, Malawi was hit by the Cashgate scandal in which US$31 million had been stolen from government coffers. A total of one-third of government funds have been stolen in the last ten years. This has led to a withdrawal of many sources of foreign aid.[4] In Malawi, the "glitter of the sun rising across the lake" — its namesake — is hard to see.

Papua New Guinea, 2009

Who were the leaders? In our work in Papua New Guinea, Jens, ill and struggling with chemo treatments, was leading from a hospital bed in another country. I was his deputy, managing the team with his indirect support. Anna Irumai, the head of the Independent Monitoring and Review Group at the National Department of Health, was leading us barefoot from her desk. Ruben, the Papua New Guinean district family health coordinator, was leading with a merry smile. They were trying to strengthen and catalyze local, national, and regional leadership to solve overwhelming problems. But the power was in the hands of others, clever and capable Papua New Guineans who were siphoning off money in a tight, enmeshed *wantok*.

We reported directly to Anna. She was sitting in her office, shaking her head and frowning. "This province isn't doing well. We follow simple things to see how they're managing — what percentage of women deliver in the health facility, how many children under one are immunized, death rates of children under five from pneumonia. We don't know why they're having problems. Is it bad management? Are they misusing the money? Very little of the money is getting out to the health facilities or outreach patrols. Please get out there and see what's going on."

Anna assigned Mark, Yvonne, and me to visit another poor province that wasn't doing well. She gave each of us a hug. "Give Jens my love when you talk to him. Tell him we miss him and we want him healthy for the next trip in six months. He knows how tough the politics are here. So he needs to get his strength back and then come here to help us."

We spent six extra hours waiting in the Port Moresby airport for our flight. Two planes had been grounded for mechanical reasons, causing delays and rescheduling. The airport seethed with patient passengers, used to the frequent delays. Those travelling to the cooler Highlands had heavy parkas, some in camouflage patterns, while other passengers sported bright fleeces in red, blue, or green. The women wore the fleeces over printed *meri* dresses (loose women's clothing that can be worn before, during, and after pregnancy). Tossed over their shoulders were crocheted bags called *bilums* in various sizes and exuberant designs of chevrons and stripes.

Children ran squealing around the waiting room with runny noses and bare feet, even if they had parkas on. One ancient woman sat on her haunches, her dirty bare feet on the floor. Her teeth were stained red from betel juice; the two top front ones were broken. She grinned mischievously. The old woman belonged in another century, with her wrinkled face and traditional tattoos on her face and arms. Yet she talked into a cellphone that she had on speaker mode, using it like a microphone and staring at it quizzically from time to time.

We were finally loaded into the plane, and after a two-hour ride were greeted by a welcoming party from the provincial health department. Ruben explained that since we were travelling in the rainy season it was easier to move by boat on the swollen rivers (so the dinghy wouldn't hit rocks), rather than on the rough open sea, where the risk of drowning was high and life jackets were seldom available. Two people had drowned the week before trying to bring a woman with a complicated delivery to the hospital.

To reach the boat for our journey by river we had to cross from the wharf to the shore, but the bridge had washed out. High above the water there was now an impromptu footbridge — two very narrow, flattened logs connected to a ten-square-foot platform, another fifteen feet to the next platform, and so on for a total of four sections. There was barely space to place one sandal-clad foot on each log. The other side looked impossibly far away.

I watched the slender logs bend and sway under Mark's and Ruben's weight. Then I looked at my pile of papers and my handbag, and worried about the need to balance with both of my arms. I accepted Mark's offer as he reached back to carry my reports. Ruben held out his hand. "Come on, I'll help you." He led me across the shaky surface to the first landing. As I followed them over three more sections, I thought to myself, *this really is how it is.* Often, as external health consultants we think that our technical assistance has us in the leading role. It was good to be reminded that I was following, watching, and learning in this new culture and environment, which was so challenging. I tried not to look down. Behind me, Yvonne walked with ease and graceful balance. Finally, we jumped down, barefoot, to the river shore and the squelching mud flats that oozed between our toes. We rinsed off our feet at the dinghy and greeted our boat driver. When we looked up at the storm clouds above, we knew the return journey would be wet.

The serpentine Marua River wound through tropical rainforest. Palm trees stretched as high as several-storey buildings, while vines with leaves as broad as my arm curved up their trunks. In some areas mangroves grew, sheltering sago trees, the source of a staple food. On the shore we could see women making the sago, and we stopped to watch. Two ten-foot-long trees had been cut open and laid diagonally on a brace. The women scooped and pounded the inner pulp. River water was poured into the mash continually so that a thick orange liquid sieved through a leaf/rush funnel into a dugout container at the bottom of the sluice. Two women, two sago trees, the pounding in unison. By tomorrow the amber liquid would harden into a thick, crusty porridge ready to be cooked into a crumbly biscuit. I was intrigued at the capacity for survival. The nourishing secrets of an unlikely looking tree, and such a complicated way to convert it to food, had been discovered over generations of living close to the land. Mostly carbohydrate, sago was usually eaten like a pancake with fish.

As I watched, the thoughts I'd had while crossing the river coalesced. Developing countries can, and must, lead the process of change. Local communities have, and use, knowledge that has helped them survive.

My PNG counterparts were my leaders. Ruben knew the local situation, and Anna, at the national level, was trying to point us in the right direction so that we might uncover misused funding in a poor, struggling province. She had the knowledge of what was going on in her country, since she followed all the health indicators and analyzed the strengths and weaknesses of each province and district. But she lacked the political power to challenge the corruption she could see. For this she needed partners such as us to bring the weight of donor countries from the outside to help in her struggle with corrupt leaders.

Anna was technically excellent. She had set up a monitoring system backed by an Australian epidemiologist named Michael Douglas and supported by global experts on maternal health, such as Wendy Graham, from Edinburgh, to help track the faltering progress or declines in goals such as improved poverty and death rates of mothers and children. When we visited this province at her request, we did find examples of misused money, of salaries that hadn't been paid, of health workers who couldn't do their jobs because of obstruction by their leaders. But even joining our voice with Anna's, we lacked the political power to challenge the leaders in her country. National leaders with political power may be motivated by their own personal greed and can easily silence those who try to lead a process of change for improved health.

GHANA, 1997

"Don't you trust me? I'm the chief thief." So said the man who had been carefully sought out by my pregnant Canadian friend living in Ghana. She worked in mother-and-child health in a poor rural region of the country. She had lost a stereo, a computer, a printer, and other belongings from both her home and office. The informal communication channels had involved a soothsayer and a repentant young man who was responsible for part of the theft. Now the chief thief had been asked to intervene.

Each town in Ghana had a chief thief. "Retired" from the business, he still oversaw the division of spoils. He knew who had stolen what and from whom. If asked to intervene, he decided whether to extend his protection to the victim or to the perpetrator of the crime. In my friend's case, he decided in her favour because of her good work with the poor. And he had children himself. He didn't feel right allowing a pregnant woman to be exploited by thieves. Therefore he was obliged to withdraw his protection from the thief and inform on him.

A police raid of the thief's home revealed nothing (on account of a bribe paid to the police by the thief's family), but again the informal channels resulted in all the goods being returned to their rightful owner.

Meanwhile, my friend tried to arrange schooling and a job for the young man, who now showed remorse and admitted his part in the theft. When a group of colleagues discussed this case, other examples were shared. One Ghanaian midwife from another town told us her mother, who was also a midwife, delivered the baby of the chief thief and received lifelong protection from theft.

We, in the affluent West, have become the chief thieves. But we have been less successful in protecting pregnant women than this Ghanaian chief thief.

In 1997 the flow of resources between rich and poor countries was even. Poor countries now give money to rich ones. Even Sub-Saharan Africa is now a money exporter. In 2006 the net transfer of capital from poorer countries to rich ones (United Nations data) was $784 billion, up from $229 billion in 2002.[5] Complicated mathematical formulae describe and explain this phenomenon — the Lucas Paradox.[6]

Developing countries borrow (for armies to ensure their leaders live in affluence) and then have huge debts to pay back, requiring them to cut back on social spending, health, education for the poor, and wages for workers in the social sectors. The poor wages available for health workers cause them to flee to wealthier countries that are actively recruiting them. The poorest parts of poor countries can never compete. There are fewer health workers where the needs are greatest. In many Third World countries you can draw regional maps plotting inversely high under-five child mortality rates and increased deaths of pregnant women, with low nurse/midwife per capita ratios. The poor have higher child and maternal mortality rates, as well as the least access to skilled health workers.

More than 40 percent of college-educated people in much of Africa are actively recruited by the United Kingdom and other English-speaking nations; they immigrate to rich countries so that now two-thirds of nursing posts in Malawi's public health system are vacant.[7]

Malawi is one of several countries in the world with a death rate of over 1,000 pregnant women per 100,000 live births.[8] Zambia has lost three-quarters of its new physicians in recent years. Even in South Africa, more than one-fifth of graduating doctors migrate. But this trend costs South Africa the one hundred thousand dollars per physician it spends to train a doctor.[9] This huge and widening gap in human resources limits the ability to fight infectious diseases or to deliver babies safely.

An external brain drain takes away skilled midwives to other countries: there is currently a global shortage of 350,000 midwives, with severe shortages in seventy countries with high maternal and child mortality rates.[10] An internal brain drain takes them from delivering babies to other better paying roles, such as HIV prevention and treatment for which they might earn three times their usual wage. The most debt-affected countries have also implemented systems of cost recovery for health care, making safe delivery and emergency obstetric care unaffordable for poor women. The widest discrepancy between the poor and the rich is seen in maternal health services.[11] In this context it isn't surprising that the death rate of delivering women has shown little progress in regions such as Sub-Saharan Africa.

The world tried to respond. *The Lancet* medical journal highlighted the problem of maternal deaths in a special series in 2006.[12] An extra $10.2 billion dollars is needed annually to save six million maternal and neonatal lives. In 2006, $3.5 billion was spent, one-third of the needs. A global conference on delivering women, Deliver Now, was held in the United Kingdom in 2007 and established a partnership for maternal, neonatal, and child health.[13] In late 2007 the prime minister of Norway committed $1 billion over the next ten years and created a network of global leaders to work to address the inequities in maternal health. Philanthropic organizations such as the Bill and Melinda Gates Foundation and the Buffett Foundation have committed resources for maternal health.

In March 2008 a Maternal Health Parliamentarian Forum in the United Kingdom highlighted the need for urgent political commitment. Plans were made to strengthen health systems, address the crisis in human resources, and provide effective technologies to deliver such drugs as magnesium sulfate for pre-eclampsia and misoprostol for hemorrhaging. Policies were discussed to subsidize maternal health care with different health-financing initiatives. Action was mobilized with the G8 and other leaders to support civil society groups such as the White Ribbon Alliance against maternal death and the International Planned Parenthood Federation to ensure access to contraceptives. Wider issues were also addressed such as investments in female education, integration of HIV care in maternal health services, and the strengthening of services for adolescents.

Examples were given such as Sri Lanka, which had removed all user fees and now had 95 percent of women delivering with a skilled midwife. Uganda and some districts in Zambia had increased utilization of maternal health services when user fees were abolished. Ghana was convinced to pay for maternal health in its National Health Insurance Scheme, using funds from the U.K. government (through budget support, or non-earmarked money that could be allocated to any sector), though contraceptive services still weren't paid for. Other successful models were cited such as Nepal, which saw a halving of maternal deaths when access to skilled attendants, emergency obstetric care, family planning, and safe abortion was improved.[14]

The U.K. Parliamentary Forum criticized the fragmented leadership of the United Nations, which had complicated support for maternal health and advocated for better synergy of UN initiatives.

The forum also raised the concern about financing for maternal health: less than one-tenth of the money needed for maternal and neonatal health had been mobilized, eclipsed by HIV spending. For example, the U.K. Parliamentary Enquiry on Maternal Health, published in October 2007, found that in 2004 the United Kingdom raised $62 million for maternal and neonatal health, but in 2004–7 it raised $3 billion for HIV. The United Kingdom gives one dollar per person a year for the health of mothers and their newborns — half of that contributed by Norway, but five times more than American or Japanese citizens contribute.

Some countries responded with united support for maternal health. In Canada, in June 2009, Jim Abbott, parliamentary secretary to the minister of international co-operation, introduced an all-party resolution, which was passed unanimously. It read: "That this House renews its commitment to reducing maternal and newborn morbidity and mortality both at home and abroad and supports Canadian leadership within government and civil society to work within the G8 and as partners with UN agencies and appropriate global initiatives to achieve this goal."[15]

A follow-up global conference in 2010 informed the G8 Summit on the latest strategies to improve maternal health. Technical, political, and grassroots leaders, including women with maternal morbidities such as obstetric fistula, told the world it was time to change. Plans were made to save these lives by providing simple, low-cost primary health-care interventions, similar to the success that had been achieved in saving two million lives from infectious diseases by resources mobilized by the Global Fund.

In 2010, U.S. President Barack Obama unveiled the Global Health Initiative, which doubled American funding for maternal and child health.[16] It was easier for the United States to come up with a $700 billion bailout for highly paid Wall Street gamblers, but we haven't raised the $10.2 billion that is needed annually to save the lives of six million pregnant women and newborn infants.[17] Who will work for the nearly ten million pregnant women, their newborns, and their children under five who die every year in the developing world?[18] Who will work for the up to ten million more women who will become disabled because of pregnancy complications?[19]

Ninety percent of these women and infants live, for their short, tragic lives, in South Asia and Sub-Saharan Africa. In Sub-Saharan Africa all mothers face the risk that one out of sixteen pregnant women will die.[20]

There has been some momentum in improving maternal health globally.[21] This is an opportunity for cautious optimism. However, in some countries, such as Zimbabwe, Nigeria, and Papua New Guinea, the situation has worsened. This is also the case even in developed countries like the United States and Canada. Globally, the vast majority of the poor are still hugely unserved.

It was estimated that $200 billion (of which $5 billion annually is to reduce maternal deaths) would be needed by 2015 to reduce poverty and maternal and child death rates, to improve the status of women, and to limit infectious diseases, including AIDS.

Why is it so hard to put the last first?

How is it possible, for example, that in Papua New Guinea, where the economy is growing and development spending has risen dramatically, that the death rates of pregnant women have doubled from 1996 to 2006 so that one woman in twenty-five will die during pregnancy?[22]

What are we doing wrong, and how can we get it right?

All development partners are locked into political dynamics. When the George W. Bush government blocked funding in 2002 to the United Nations Population Fund over its refusal to ban funding for abortion, other donors managed to make up for that lost money.[23] The money withheld by the U.S. government would have been enough to save 250,000 women's lives.

To meet the global target to reduce maternal mortality by three-quarters by 2015, death rates of pregnant women needed to drop more than 5 percent a year. Instead, the annual decline was 2.3 percent, not on track to meet the Millennium Development Goal of improving maternal health.[24] What is going to happen during the current financial collapse where wealthy governments are bailing out wealthy banks using taxpayers' money?

Many poor countries have started to reduce death rates for children. For example, in Tanzania in 2006 the country already exceeded its planned reductions in the death rates of infants and children, with drops from 20 to 40 percent in ten years.[25] But progress in maternal health plateaued. In Bangladesh by 2000, death rates for children achieved impressive declines up to 40 percent, a momentum that has continued to improve, but maternal health also stalled.[26] Ghana is well on the way to middle-income status, but there is little progress in reducing maternal deaths in the poorest parts of the nation, and the gap between rich and poor is widening.[27] In all of these countries, governments have tried to put maternal health on the agenda but have had difficulty mobilizing money, prioritizing these resources, and deploying the health workers necessary to build a sustainable system.

What happens when there are such gaps between rich and poor? How can this be turned around? The world has created an economic system that encourages borrowing beyond one's means in an elusive search for status. In many countries where I work, poor young women, schoolgirls, don't think of themselves as prostitutes. But they do admit to trading sex with older, married, and richer boyfriends for top-up time on their cellphones. Intergenerational transactional sex is a major factor in the HIV epidemic, and teenage pregnancies are a major factor in maternal deaths. Unless we have stronger strategies to address gender and income differentials, it will be a slow process to transform maternal health outcomes.

Such a strange juxtaposition of cultures makes up the global partnership. Our current development work is a complex form of cross-cultural confusion.

At the time of first contact between Papua New Guinea and white settlers in search of resources such as minerals and oil, the whites hired planes to drop provisions for them from the air — food, bedding, clothing, furniture, cooking utensils, and tools. The local tribes found this astonishing. What god was this who dropped gifts from the sky? Thinking these white people had a powerful religion, many PNG natives sought conversion to Christianity. But some created "cargo cults." They, too, built airstrips and waited, hoping that the new gods would see them and drop presents from the sky.

Development has become a new cargo cult. We, too, are dropping money from the sky. We are poised with our largesse — millions of dollars to combat HIV/AIDS, tuberculosis, malaria, and other forms of ill health. Instead of airstrips, we have built complicated accounting forms and management systems that have also contributed to corruption. Instead, we have to build systems designed to ensure the money gets down to the ground where it is most needed and where the least visible goal, improving maternal health, can also receive attention.

Only five wealthy countries have met their commitment to give 0.7 percent of their GDP to development aid.[28] In meetings in Abuja, Nigeria, African countries committed to spend 15 percent of their government allocation to the health sector, largely to address HIV/AIDS and malaria. But the failure to meet the Abuja commitment has also further squeezed funding for maternal and neonatal health.

The 2010 G8 Summit put maternal health on the agenda, with $7.3 billion committed over the next five years for mother-and-child health, $5 billion of which was from G8 countries and the remainder from private foundations and non-G8 countries and organizations (Netherlands, Norway, New Zealand, South Korea, Spain, Switzerland, the Gates Foundation, and the UN Foundation). Over $10 billion had been anticipated by NGOs and other development partners; some even hoped for $20 billion over the next five years. One-fifth of the new money pledged was committed by Canada, the G8 host, at the Muskoka Initiative[29] (equal to the cost to Canada of hosting the G8/G20 Summits), giving limited new momentum to the UN-led Joint Action Plan to Improve the Health of Women and Children. But within these pledges, political uncertainty rested on what would be funded. Canada declined to fund abortion and limited access to family planning. Family planning remains the most cost-effective way to save women's lives. Money hasn't been mobilized in sufficient quantities to train and deploy midwives, especially in Sub-Saharan Africa, and skilled attendants at delivery remains a crucial requirement to save women's lives in pregnancy.

Other initiatives followed. There have been complementary efforts. Christy Turlington Burns made the movie *No Woman, No Cry* after suffering pregnancy complications. She filmed in Tanzania, Guatemala, Bangladesh, and the United States, and also created the organization Every Mother Counts. That organization has "sponsor midwife training" programs and runs a program to equip health-care workers in South Sudan.[30]

Johnson & Johnson has a program called Saving Mothers' and Babies' Lives. It has partnered with UNICEF/Safe Motherhood Initiative to provide technical support and training programs to midwives, female health workers, and staff nurses in Madya Pradesh and Rajasthan, India. The number of institutional deliveries in these provinces has increased from 35 percent in 2004 to 76 percent in 2007. They provide twenty-four-hour care.[31]

The Maternal Health Thematic Fund was created in 2008 to improve progress in the world's poorest countries because improving maternal health is the slowest Millennium Development Goal. The fund works to strengthen midwifery and emergency obstetric care, contraceptive and reproductive commodities availability, and the Campaign to End Fistula. As of December 2010, the fund had received more than $60 million in donations. It has given assistance in thirty countries, and an additional twelve have received support for an obstetric fistula program.

We have leadership, and this must be further consolidated to strengthen impact. And we have to have strategies to work with corrupt countries that have abdicated their leadership or replaced action with talk, so we don't hear the lament from poor, suffering women: "Where are our leaders? Why have they forgotten us?"

When a pregnant woman is in labour, the progress is best followed with a partograph. This is a tool for watchful waiting. It has two lines: an alert one and an action one. The alert line shows that progress isn't on track. The action line dictates that intervention is needed such as emergency obstetric care. World leaders have agreed we aren't on track to reduce the deaths of pregnant women and their newborn children, and that we need to commit to action. We have crossed the alert line.

We are still waiting to see if the right actions will be taken.

We Are Still Waiting:

Bangladesh, Laos, and Nigeria

Bangladesh, 2010

Sultana's grin was infectious, and she laughed joyfully. She joked about her former husband and his new wife and children. "Maybe I will sew dresses for his daughters!" She chuckled. Unable to bear children herself, she held no bitterness for the husband who had abandoned her after her own baby boy had been stillborn three years earlier. Nor did she seem angry about the tearing from the obstructed labour that created a fistula requiring eight operations to repair.

"We didn't know any better then," she told me. "My mother was with me. She delivered all of us safely at home."

We were a team of five — Dr. Mizan and Dr. Shirin, who were Bangladeshis; Dr. Marta Medina and I, who were public health doctors; and Dr. Thomas Raassen, a fistula repair surgeon who looked surprisingly like Jens Hasfeldt. I had worked with Marta in several countries; she had met Jens Hasfeldt in Nicaragua and had joined his group in Copenhagen. It felt good that we were carrying on the work we had both shared with Jens.

Sultana was dressed in her finest and held two red roses in her hands, which picked up the red trim on her sari. She was seated with five young

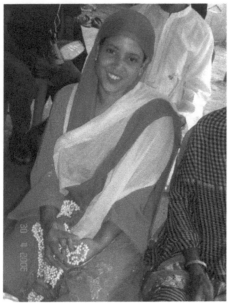

Sultana, a fistula survivor, in Bangladesh.

women in their early teens whom she was teaching to sew at her own tailoring shop, down a muddy path from her own home. Her parents also sat with her, her father distinguished in white, with a fine greying beard, and her mother who struggled with tears as she told us how the family had sacrificed to pay for the operations. "We sold our goats, our water buffalo, the rice paddies, that piece of land over there that has now been built upon by our neighbour for his son. Even though the surgery was free, so many other costs! Transport to the hospitals, paying for food for the family members who accompanied her. But she is well now. I cried the first day I brought her home and there was no leaking of urine in her bed. I cried because we were happy."

Sultana was mature for her twenty years. She had gathered her community around her small shop filled with items for sale: neat racks of carefully sewn children's outfits, pillowcases, handkerchiefs. Her shop was an open stall with an awning overhead to protect it from the rain. Roosters pecked hopefully for grains of food in the sand around the store. It had taken us an hour by rickshaw through the squelching mud and light drizzle, the rickshaw *wallahs* pedalling and straining with the effort, to reach her village. Sultana was explaining things to the villagers gathered around her, men in one row and women of all ages in the other. "It is best to give birth in the clinic, or have the community-skilled birth attendant come to you at home. Don't deliver with the *dai,* or the village quack. You know my story. You know that by the time we realized the baby wouldn't come, it was too late to get help." She asked each woman in turn where they would have their babies. The older ones, mothers already and dressed in their best saris — a bright bouquet of peach, magenta, cool green, and blue — shyly peeked out from behind their veils and said that they would still prefer to deliver at home. The young unmarried girls, just home from school and casually dressed in smart *shalwar kameezes,* all chose a health facility delivery. The men listened carefully as the rain pattered on the tin roof above our heads.

Sultana was now a community fistula advocate, using her own difficult experience to convince other women to deliver safely. In simple language she explained how to detect when the labour was prolonged, where to go for help, what a fistula was, and how it could be repaired.

She wanted to share her good fortune. "I have been helped. I was given money to start my shop. I could help other women with this problem. I could teach them to sew. I will encourage them if the first operations aren't successful. I can help here in my community. Other women like me have told the world about this problem. I have learned that other fistula survivors have spoken out in England and America. They have helped get more attention to prevent and treat this problem of fistula by making sure women get good care when they are delivering."[1] Sultana's grin was infectious, and she laughed joyfully.

All over Bangladesh there are only about five hundred operations to repair obstetric fistulas that can be performed every year. But at least ten times more women will develop fistulas each year, since only 10 percent of women have supervised births by a skilled birth attendant and less than 2 percent have access to emergency obstetric care. And over seventy thousand women in Bangladesh already have fistulas. Most of those women don't have access to community fistula advocates like Sultana to understand the treatment or can't afford to get to care even if they know about the possibility of repair.[2]

Despite support from the United Nations and NGOs to care for women with fistula and to try to prevent women from developing this problem, too many women are still waiting. In the Democratic Republic of the Congo about one-third of new cases are repaired, but the backlog is over forty thousand. Many of those fistulas are from traumatic rape, women who have been victims in the civil war. In Nigeria just over two thousand repairs are done every year, but there are twenty thousand new cases and a backlog of more than two hundred thousand cases. In Pakistan less than four hundred repairs are done every year, but over ten times more cases develop each year. In Sudan only a couple of hundred repairs are done every year, but five thousand new cases occur each year because of the lack of maternity care for displaced women in Darfur and nearby war-torn regions.[3]

One of the lucky ones was Chandra. She was a little shy, but she was the spokesperson for her group of eight women. Although they had been waiting for at least three months, they would be getting surgery. In the meantime they were receiving lessons in reading and numbers while they waited. "Each of us has been able to choose a skill for training — sewing, cooking, raising animals, growing vegetables," explained Chandra. The Bangladesh Women's Health Coalition organized their lessons and ran the residence where they could stay with their children while they had preoperative investigations and waited for a date for surgery to repair their fistulas, which had torn their genitals into their bladder or rectum, due to unsupervised obstructed labour. "All of us lost our last babies. They were all born dead. But that was three or four years ago for all of us. It has taken us that long to learn we have fistulas, to understand they can be treated, to raise the money to get to a hospital, and to be referred here for surgery."

Chandra had a six-year-old daughter named Chitta. She had been born safely. But her second child was a boy who was a little bigger. That slightly larger child was a more difficult birth. "I had my baby at home. I had no money to pay for a midwife or to go to the hospital. I had a *dai*. I could pay her with a sari. But she didn't realize I was having problems, and after I was in labour for twenty-two hours, she said I needed to go to the hospital. But I had no money, and we had no way to get there. So I kept trying to give birth at home. Six hours later my son was born dead, but I had torn badly inside. I didn't know what was wrong. I kept leaking urine, which was smelly. No one wanted me to stay with them. My husband left. I was alone with my daughter. We had no money. I couldn't work; I couldn't chip bricks for gravel. My family helped me a little. My parents took me back to live with them. Then I met Sultana. She told me I could be helped. She had needed eight different surgeries to become well. I am afraid. I hope I will be cured with one operation."

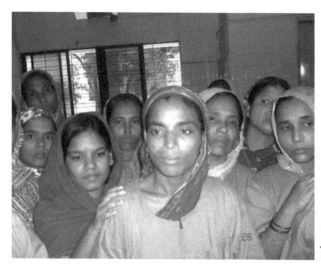

*Women in
Bangladesh wait
for their fistula
repairs.*

She smiled. "We are still waiting, but we are waiting with hope. We understand that the surgeons can't get time in the operating room to help us, since they don't make money. And we understand it is a costly, long surgery. And we understand there are few doctors who do this work." Chandra smiled again, a bright, beaming grin, and took the hand of Chitta. "We are waiting with hope because we know we are leading. Others will follow. We are making the path for them." She gazed at Chitta. "She won't suffer as I have."

The next day our same team travelled to another village in a Hindu settlement near Kumudini Hospital. Here we met a community-skilled birth attendant (CSBA),[4] one of five thousand in the country who have been trained in the past two years to deliver women at home using a partograph to monitor their labour and with medicines for pre-eclampsia and hemorrhage. She was proud with her white lab coat over her simple sari, a stethoscope peeking out of her pocket. The CSBA, too, explained to a cheerful crowd of twenty or so women seated on jute mats on the ground about the prevention of obstructed labour and other warning signs such as prolonged bleeding after birth. She answered the questions of the women, then said she wanted us to come with her. Thomas Raassen was still in surgery, assessing the quality of the fistula repair team at Kumudini Hospital, so Marta, Mizan, Shirin, and I followed her into a wood-and-mud home in the compound. A young mother sat shyly in a blue cotton sari on a bed with her newborn,

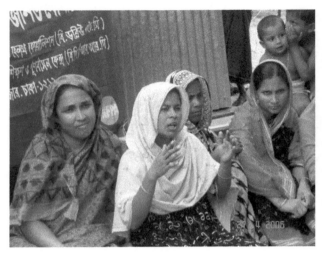

A community fistula advocate in Bangladesh advises other women how to prevent fistula by having a supervised delivery.

delivered the day before. The CSBA showed us the partograph, which she had completed carefully to show how well the labour had progressed. "I have delivered eighty-five babies this year. And it is only Ramadan. I will deliver many more in the next four months." The young mother glanced up at the CSBA, smiled, and started to suckle her baby.

We stepped out of the home, and I began to weep. Mizan rushed over to see what the matter was. "Like Sultana's mother, I'm crying because I'm happy. It's been such a long journey, so much work, to get to this place where women can deliver with the supports of home, but with the midwifery skills to manage births safely."

Laos, 2012

Moving quickly into middle income status, Laos, or Lao People's Democratic Republic (Lao PDR), is a challenge with wide inequities in access to reproductive, maternal, and child health between income groups, and rural indigenous people being particularly disadvantaged. In addition, the country is largely dependent on external health financing. The WHO, in its strategy for the Asia Pacific Region, suggests that 4–5 percent of government expenditures should be directed towards health. In 2011–12, the year of our evaluation in Laos, 3.7 percent of domestic expenditures went to the health sector, behind Cambodia and Vietnam at around 9 percent and Thailand at over 14 percent.[5] In terms of the new global objectives of sustainable development goals, dependence on external donors needs to be lessened.

The legacy of the Communist era is felt in the need to make toasts with vodka at every opportunity such as visiting small clinics or hospitals and meeting with elected officials, a skill I tried to master. This added a slightly surreal feeling as we travelled to remote settlements, which have a majority of the indigenous people and the fewest health services.

Development assistance can help direct support to unmet needs. Our evaluation of financing from Luxemburg Development to health was positive in terms of monies allocated to poor provinces with large indigenous populations, and to training of midwives from those ethnic minorities, to help increase skilled birth attendants for those underserved regions. In addition, a voucher scheme had been designed to benefit those in the hardest to reach communities, so that women and children under five in those villages would be able to access preventive and curative care. Vouchers are ways that underserved vulnerable groups can get health care and transport to services paid for by national governments or donors so this does not become an out-of-pocket expense that would be unaffordable for the poor. The project had also used its experience to help design a draft National Health Financing Strategy to help operationalize free maternal health care and treatment for children under five, a national initiative starting in over forty of the poorest districts in the country. Health workers from the poorest and most remote regions (ethnic minorities) also received support from the project to upgrade skills.

In 2018, Laos was cited as the third most unequal country in terms of access to reproductive, maternal, newborn, child, and adolescent health (RMNCAH),[6] using 2011 data. Nigeria had the greatest inequity, followed by Angola. These findings were based on composite indicators of coverage encompassing the continuum of RMNCAH care, which are being tracked as part of the Countdown to 2030:[7]

- *Pre-pregnancy* (satisfied demand for family planning with modern methods);
- *Pregnancy care* (at least four prenatal visits including for adolescents aged 15–19, intermittent preventive treatment for malaria among

pregnant women, anti-retroviral therapy for pregnant women living with HIV, and neonatal tetanus protection);

- *Birth* (skilled attendant at birth including for adolescents aged 15–19, total public and private health facility births; and total urban and rural Caesarean sections);
- *Postnatal care* (for all mothers including adolescents aged 15–19, their babies, and early initiation of breastfeeding);
- *Infancy* (exclusive breastfeeding under six months, continued breastfeeding 12–15 months, three doses of immunization against diphtheria, pertussis, and tetanus (DPT3) and oral polio, first dose of measles vaccine, three doses of pneumococcal vaccine, and rotavirus immunization);
- *Childhood* (two doses of Vitamin A supplementation, children under five sleeping under insecticide-treated nets, malaria diagnostics for children under five, care seeking for acute respiratory infection, oral rehydration salts for diarrhea, oral rehydration salts plus zinc for diarrhea);
- *Environment* (population using basic drinking water services, population using basic sanitation services, population sleeping under insecticide-treated nets or in a house with indoor residual spraying).

Laos had made poverty alleviation a major policy focus, and there have been significant efforts to map poverty that have helped to direct development efforts. There has also been a substantial support for immunization coverage, a key indicator, with DPT3 coverage rising from 42 to 53 percent and increases in tetanus immunization for pregnant women to reduce neonatal tetanus from 2009 to 2011, the period we were evaluating. The project had also helped to improve the health management information system, to enable tracking of system achievements. These are all important initiatives, and it will be interesting to continue to monitor the progress of achieving equity in RMNCAH in the Lao People's Democratic Republic.

Other countries with indigenous populations have faced similar challenges, including developed countries such as Canada. In 2009 leaders of the Society of Obstetricians and Gynecologists of Canada raised concerns about maternal health in Indigenous communities in Canada.

Living in more isolated areas and with other socio-economic factors affecting maternal health, Indigenous women in Canada had higher rates

COMPARISON OF INDIGENOUS AND NON-INDIGENOUS MATERNAL HEALTH INDICATORS		
	Indigenous	**Non-Indigenous**
Mothers under age 18	9 percent	1 percent
Post-neonatal deaths **One month to one year**	6.85 per 1,000 live births	2.1 per 1,000 live births
Infant mortality rate	12.0 per 1,000 live births	6 per 1,000 live births
Spousal homicide rate[a]	4.72 per 100,000 couples	0.58 per 100,000 couples

Source: Lalonde, Butt, and Bucio, *JOGC*, October 2009.
[a]Gender-based violence is a major determinant of maternal health.

of maternal death, and the policy of evacuating women to be delivered by non-Indigenous health workers in health facilities had undermined the cultural supports for delivering women. A policy was developed to help train indigenous midwives, to return birthing to communities with a multi-disciplinary, collaborative primary maternity care model following examples such as the Rankin Inlet Birthing Centre and Irnisuksiiniq-Inuit Midwifery Network. Similarly Chile, Bolivia, Argentina, Peru among other countries, have attempted to integrate culturally supportive models of skilled birth attendants for indigenous minorities.

Laos, therefore, is not alone in facing these challenges of equity for reproductive, maternal, newborn, and child health for rural ethnic minorities. Developed and developing countries share both these difficulties and the potential strategies for change.

NIGERIA, 2015

While half of mothers in Nigeria received at least four antenatal care visits, there were wide equity gaps by education and geography as well as in the status of women. Only 38 percent (a negligible rise from 35.2 percent in 2003) of births in Nigeria were delivered by a skilled health provider such as a midwife, doctor, or nurse, but 67 percent of urban women had access to skilled attendants at delivery compared to 23 percent of rural mothers.

Forty percent of women received a postnatal visit within two days of delivery, but, again, there were wide regional and socio-economic variations.[8]

Income inequality drives the inequity in access to MNCH services. Nigeria was off track to meet the 2015 targets for Millennium Development Goals 4 and 5, to reduce child mortality and improve maternal health. But what of the shift to the Sustainable Development Goals with their greater focus on adolescent health, sustainability, and equity? According to the 2013 DHS, younger adolescents in Nigeria aged 15–17 have lower rates of satisfied demand for family planning (27 percent), four prenatal visits (31 percent), and skilled birth attendant (22 percent), compared to women 20–49 years of age (36 percent, 53 percent and 40 percent, respectively). A user pay system will make it hard to address these gaps.

In Nigeria, 7 percent of total government expenditure is allocated to health, but out-of-pocket expenditure by Nigerians is 66 percent of total health expenditure, which leads to wide inequities in access to health services by income quintile. This is a time for concern in Nigeria. Many countries are reducing their development aid to Nigeria because of challenges in their own economies, or for political reasons such as the current American policies against family planning and reproductive health including adolescent health.

The country has a population of over 160 million and ranks poorly (153 out of 187) on the Human Development Index (HDI); 65 percent of the population lives below the poverty line. The maternal mortality ratio is 576 deaths per 100,000 live births. One in eight Nigerian children will die before the age of five. Over half a million children die every year from three leading preventable illnesses: pneumonia, diarrhea, and malaria. In 2011, less than 45 percent of infants had been immunized with three doses against diphtheria, polio, tetanus, and pertussis, and HIV rates were increasing. The coverage to prevent mother-to-child transmission of HIV with anti-retroviral drugs is decreasing. The country is off-track to meet the goal of access to safe water, and the coverage of sanitation services is falling rather than rising.

Nigeria is one of three countries (with Pakistan and Afghanistan) in the world that still has polio, particularly in the north of the country. The continued focus on monitoring progress towards the Sustainable Development Goals will help keep these issues in focus both within Nigeria and with its development partners.

Endings:

Papua New Guinea, Tanzania, Bhutan, and a Global Reflection

Another world is not only possible, she's on the way and, on a quiet day, if you listen very carefully you can hear her breathe.
—Arundhati Roy

Papua New Guinea, 2009

We were staying in a guest house with a huge wood fire to warm us against the cold. It was a cold night, typical for the Highlands. A police guard stayed with us in the house; there was a state of emergency nearby, close to a mine. At noon the smell of roasting pig, with a sweet overlay of edible ferns, drifted out from the large cooking pit where the pig was being prepared for our welcome feast. Several whole chickens and fifty potatoes and twenty sweet potatoes were also baking over hot coals. The potatoes had been presented to us in a large *bilum*, a woven or crocheted bag of varying size in which anything from a baby to large sacks of vegetables can be carried.

The courtyard in front of the upgraded health centre still awaited a maternity section for women to deliver their babies. So far it lacked water, had few medicines, and possessed only Tylenol for the pain of labour. There was ergometrine for control of bleeding after delivery; the previous month there had been none. There was no light source. The week before, a baby who had been born on the cold concrete floor in the dark died. Not surprisingly, only three women had delivered here in the past four weeks. The one community health worker was a man. Few women would be comfortable being delivered by him; their husbands wouldn't allow it.

It was raining in the courtyard as I heard stories of the deaths. We sat on the ground in clearings under the trees, the villagers unmindful of the rain. The village health worker was eloquent. He wore yellow marigolds decoratively over each ear, and a festive sprig of green fern crowned his head as he told us about his wife and newborn child who had both died here the year before. There were no medicines, radio to call for help, or ambulance, nothing to stop the convulsions that ended his young wife's short life.

Another woman came to the centre of the clearing to talk about her last child, stillborn here in the health centre. She wore a man's black coat over her meri, rain glistening on her face joining the tears she was wiping away, first with a hand over her right cheekbone, then over her left. The hundreds of people who ringed the courtyard murmured their support, shaking their heads sadly.

The rain fell heavier, but still hundreds of men, women, and children sat wetly, entranced, during the hours of speeches.

Four sad hours later I was led through squelching mud down a path dotted with clay-covered stones, through wet overhanging branches to a larger arch festooned with garlands of roses and marigolds. I was being welcomed to a maternity waiting house that the men had built of bush materials gathered by the women. Inside, a log fire kept the long earthen room, with seating and resting areas ringing it, warm and a little smoky against the cool, wet air of the Highlands.

Jens had wanted to come. He knew it would be his last trip to Papua New Guinea. I talked with him daily on Skype as he lay in his bed at home, in France. His voice was wheezy. "Just a little bronchitis. I'm on antibiotics."

I tried to laugh, joking with him about his severe allergies to all but one antibiotic, recalling the anaphylactic reaction he had suffered when a colleague on a mission with him in Africa had inadvertently prescribed something he was sensitive to. "Jens, are you sure you should be coming? What if you get sicker? And what about that wheezing? Has your doctor done a CT scan?"

I was thinking of how far his cancer had spread on our last trip together, when his doctor had stopped chemotherapy because it wasn't working. He had been very weak and had required hours of rest during the day. Our team had worked hard to keep him in a leadership role while he was so ill. That had been five months earlier.

"No, I'm good," he said. "I'll be fine. Just a little bronchitis." Worried, I called our colleagues in Belgium — Leo Deville and his wife, Martine.

"I think he's too sick. He can't do it. I can't do it. I can't be his deputy when he's this sick and still look after him. His risk is too high. Long-haul flights, cancer that's widespread, the risk of blood clots in his lung. I can't do it. It's too risky for him to be in PNG with weak medical care when he's this sick."

Jens was putting a brave face on things. He was having telephone conference calls with all the partners, with the government of Papua New Guinea, with the United Nations, with Australia, with New Zealand. He was writing the terms of reference for our mission from his bed.

I was getting increasingly upset and trying to cope with juggling my chaotic life. My schedule included Easter with my children, who were now adults themselves, up north in my home, then a meeting in New York, two days later, with the United Nations Population Fund on the evaluation of the Campaign to End Fistula. I would do that with Marta Medina, my co-team leader, who had worked with me on several continents since Jens had first introduced us in the 1990s, and we had worked together in Zambia. From New York I would go to Papua New Guinea for one month to evaluate a project designed to help pregnant women, then stay on for another month to work with Jens, continuing our review of the whole health sector.

I talked again with Leo and Martine. Maybe I should fly through France? I talked to Jens. He said, "No, don't come through France. I'll see you in PNG in another two months."

I didn't like his voice. I wasn't sure what to do. Long-distance diagnosis? I talked to Jens's wife, Diana. "He has to see a specialist." The family doctor in France finally called a chest specialist. The CT scan was done. The wheezy breathing was caused by enlarged nodes that were squeezing his lungs. His doctor started immediate chemotherapy to shrink the nodes.

After talking with my kids, I made plans to go to France for Easter. Jens spoke to me, his voice faint and rasping on the phone. "No, I realize I'm too sick to go to PNG. You can carry on. Come and see me on your way home. I'm too weak for visitors until this bronchitis clears up. Wait till you've finished in PNG, then you can tell me all about it on your way home."

Then he called and left me one last message of love and farewell. That message has been saved. I listen to it over and over. Jens died two days later, peacefully, at home. But I wasn't peaceful. I was wretched.

I struggled through Easter, my kids holding me as I kept bursting into tears. I struggled through the meetings in New York. Marta joined me in my grief. We had both lost a dear friend and colleague. We were also discouraged: the Campaign to End Fistula wasn't keeping up with even a fraction of the new cases each year; the backlog was getting worse, and the care of pregnant women wasn't improving in most countries. I struggled through the several flights to PNG, weeping quietly in my seats on the planes.

Preparing for the first assignment, I addressed the doubling of the deaths of pregnant women in PNG in the past decade.[1] I met with my colleagues at the New Zealand High Commission and the United Nations in Port Moresby. The situation in PNG was even more turbulent than usual. Riots were breaking out in major cities — fighting against Chinese nationals. Airports were being closed because of the violence. Our team was able to get out of Port Moresby on the last flight before the airport shut down.

Perhaps it was because Jens had died and was watching over my shoulder, but I was seeing death everywhere. When our Air Niugini flight landed in Wewak, the capital of East Sepik Province, a simple coffin garlanded with red ribbons was offloaded from the hold. It contained a woman who had died in labour. A tense, weeping crowd wailed in anguish, fingers locked through the fence. This was on the right side of the one-storey airport terminal. To the left, a dozen or so painted and feathered dancers sang and drummed in welcome for a group of eight white priests who had been allowed to disembark first, coming to discuss the worsening poverty in the country that was contributing to ever-higher death rates.

Then, on the road to Maprik Health Centre, an ambulance passed by, also garlanded in red, indicating it was carrying a dead body, likely another woman who had died in labour.

We were a team of three — myself; Betty, who was from Enga, a province in PNG, and who worked in public health; and Aham, who was an obstetrician from Nigeria. Our next journey took us westward. When our flight arrived in Mount Hagen, a city in Western Highlands Province, an even larger crowd roared in sorrow as the body of a young man murdered in a bar fight in Port Moresby was offloaded from the plane. Many of these people wore white mud on their faces, signifying mourning. Three women robed in black greeted the body.

A woman from the plane also alighted, greeting the mourners with a warm embrace. She was in a group of six people who had travelled from Port Moresby. The men were either in flip-flops or workboots, with dusty jeans and ball caps. One was clean-shaven and two had beards. The woman carried a *bilum* woven with the national flag and was barefoot. Above her bare feet were a lace underskirt, then a magenta skirt, and a long *meri* with ruffled short sleeves — a wild profusion of magenta, pink, and green. The friend beside her wore a seashell-patterned *meri* and a beige underskirt, and held a *bilum* with bright flame shapes in green and orange. Over her right shoulder she carried a computer bag. Another *bilum* was over her left shoulder, in which a small child about a year old peeped out. She lifted him out of the *bilum* and kissed him quietly on the forehead.

We climbed into our vehicle and drove over the rutted roads. Garlands of flowers hung from bridges and were tied to stakes along the roads. Hundreds of people walked under brightly coloured rainbow umbrellas to congregate in a square where the body would be brought to rest. Truckloads of mud-faced mourners moved slowly through the crowds.

Our team was in Enga, the last province to be created in Papua New Guinea. This province had the highest death rates of pregnant women in the nation, and PNG was a place in which the deaths of pregnant women had doubled in the past decade. We were inaugurating the maternity home, made of bush materials, adjacent to the hospital. This waiting house was a

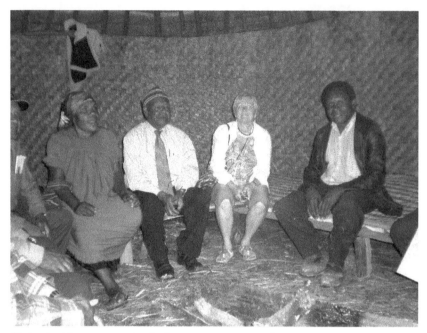

Sitting inside a community-built maternity waiting home in Enga Province,
Papua New Guinea.

community-led response to encourage mothers to come before delivery near
to the health centre, so they wouldn't face a several-hour or day-long walk in
labour through the dense bush from the high hills, only to die on the road. To
come ahead of time and stay in a homey place would bring more women close
to care. Delivery by a skilled health worker with access to emergency obstetric
care when things went wrong reduced the deaths of pregnant women. They
built these waiting homes to be ready for the upgraded delivery rooms that
had been promised years earlier by the government of PNG.

I sat on a wooden bench. Four women were telling stories in the
Enga dialect, not Tok Pisin. Betty was seated beside me and acted as my
interpreter. One woman had started to bleed before delivery and was
carried by a stretcher down the mountain to the health centre. There was
no medicine to help her, so the family had taken three hours to borrow four
hundred kina (about two hundred dollars) to hire a bus to take her to the
hospital an hour away, where she arrived dead.

Betty and I had visited that hospital and had read the list of babies born before arrival, noting how many of their mothers or the newborns, themselves, had later died. The crowded, busy ward was totally unable to hold the labouring and delivered women, who were discharged right after their babies were born. Though substandard and lacking infection prevention, a particularly difficult problem since this mining province was high in HIV infections, this hospital could at least offer a Caesarean section for emergencies.

The United Nations Population Fund had provided the region with a Jeep, and we piled into it with our bags. We moved on to another health centre still waiting for the three-year-delayed maternity upgrade, the midwives' accommodation, the medicines, and proper equipment. Here, too, the women had organized to build their own waiting house. This clearing was also dotted with hundreds of waiting people wanting to know why the construction, beds, mattresses, and equipment had been delayed.

One after the other, tearful women and angry men asked, "What happened to the plans? Where is the money? We have been told that over $300 million from oil, gold, gas, copper, nickel, and forestry development were placed in trust in a special supplementary fund. It was supposed to finance upgrading maternity wards and building midwives' accommodation in hospitals and health centres. But we have seen nothing. And now we are afraid the money has been spent on something else.[2] No one will answer our questions."

One Engan woman named Theresa called me out. "You are a white woman who has come all this way to see how we live. We didn't know that other countries were trying to help us. I am poor. I don't have the freedom you have as a woman. My own son died here in this village. We had no one to help, and there were no medicines. One day my child was running around free and playing, full of mischief. The next day he died of malaria. I have no education. Why are women dying giving life? Even my elder sister Anna died when there was no way we could stop her bleeding after the baby came. Look at the mining camps here. I am tired of seeing HIV as the price of wealth. Where are our leaders? Why have they forgotten us? We are still waiting."

She reached to the back of her neck and undid her necklace. It was made of white cowrie shells woven with black braid. She stood before me. Carefully, keeping our eyes connected, she placed it around my neck and fastened it. The value of this necklace in monetary terms couldn't be calculated. It was as though she had cut off her arm.

I spoke to her, her volunteer friends, and the other women waiting in the courtyard. "You're the most important women in Papua New Guinea," I said, my voice breaking. "You're the bravest women. You risk your lives giving life."

Back outside the maternity waiting house, Theresa stood with the other community health advocates in their blue dresses, which they had borrowed from the church choir to give themselves a special identity. The women told us what they were doing to help their communities. They stood proudly as I cut the flower ribbon and said, "This is like I am cutting the cord of a newborn baby. But cutting this cord doesn't separate us like a mother and her newborn. Cutting this cord joins us in the fight to help pregnant women deliver safely."

Our team drove on and heard singing. Ten painted men wearing feathers, grass clothing, and penis gourds stood shoulder to shoulder. I remembered Jens's story of being stopped by fighting tribesmen who had sent him away because "tomorrow we will have a war and it will not be safe." These men inched forward, chanting rhythmically, bright, curved silver spears and axes in their hands. One hundred yards away another group of men advanced, also singing. This was a compensation sing-sing.[3] Feuding between two family groups had resulted in deaths, and the two sides were now moving toward a peace agreement. Compensation (goats, pigs, cows, and kina) would be paid to the victims' families. This was the early stage of negotiation. The compensation would be paid next week. These people were prepared to compensate for the deaths they had caused, but we are still waiting for the world to pay for the maternal deaths that we are allowing to continue.

I returned to Port Moresby. In the National Department of Health, Anna Irumai stopped me outside her office and put her arms around me, crying. "We will miss him. I thought he was strong. I thought he could come for one more trip." We both wept and comforted each other, knowing Jens had left us and we would have to continue our work without him.

The head of the WHO in PNG, a Norwegian doctor named Eigil, hosted an evening gathering to welcome us, the Independent

Monitoring and Review Group. He placed a hand on my shoulder and cast a sympathetic glance. Our colleagues in the health sector in the UN agencies all missed Jens. His absence was a palpable presence that came in waves, and I felt just a little capsized. Then I looked across the room at Katja Janovsky.

Katja was elegant and professional in a chic black outfit and local shell jewellery. I hadn't seen her for a couple of years. Our last meeting had also been in Papua New Guinea — with Jens. And now here again in PNG, we met but without Jens. She had brought Jens and me together in 1989, twenty years previously, in Sudan. She crossed the room. Her face was tanned and confident. She looked much the way she had at our first meeting, in Uganda in 1987. Her glance took in my trembling lower lip, the tears threatening to fall. With no words I was folded into a firm embrace.

TANZANIA, 2015

I had last been to Tanzania for work in 2006, as team leader for the annual health sector review when we had highlighted problems in maternal health, in spite of dramatic reductions in deaths of children under one and under five. My first assignment in Tanzania had been in 1997. Then, I had worked with the government of Tanzania to help lay the groundwork for the first health sector-wide support program.

Just previous to that first assignment, while working in the U.K., I developed problems speaking. My facial creases were out of synch, and my uvula — the little thing at the back of your throat — was off-centre. I was thinking, *My mom had a stroke in her forties, with speech deficits. Me, too?* The hotel doctor referred me to a neurologist, who got me to do an MRI. No brain tumour, no MS. I paid for the investigations out of my pocket, because I really wanted to go to Tanzania, which the insurance company might not allow.

In 2015, development partners met with government to review the progress of the fourth health sector-wide program. Seeing these successes in spite of persisting challenges, I am excited I had that opportunity in 1997 to be a small part of such a positive change and that I was confident enough my health would improve to pursue that goal.

Our assignment to address the achievements in maternal and child health funded under the Canadian Muskoka Initiative coincided with a complementary team that was in-country to assess better practices in mother, newborn, and child health in four of the civil society organizations funded under the Muskoka Initiative.

How had things changed since I had been there in 2006?

In Tanzania, with a population estimated at 43 million, the estimated economic growth rate was over 7 percent per annum, and there had been continuing impressive improvements in reducing the number of deaths of children under five that was linked with decentralizing funding to the district service delivery level and providing a basic minimum package of health interventions. There had also been major supports to make insecticide-treated bed nets available to reduce malarial deaths. The country was on track to reach the millennium development goal set from 1990 to 2015, to reduce the under-five mortality rate by two-thirds with a strong immunization program, and management of childhood illnesses, including malaria and HIV.

It was not on track for reducing the newborn mortality rate (infants under twenty-eight days old) because of continued poor care for pregnant women. Only about half the women in the country had a supervised birth by a skilled birth attendant. The government's health management information system estimated in 2015 that over 60 percent of women had a facility birth; this is likely overestimated. Even in a health facility, and especially at night, women might be delivered by a medical attendant with limited skills in labour and delivery. Feedback from the civil society organizations supported by the Canadian government under the Muskoka Initiative suggested that Tanzania was not meeting the World Health Organization standards for a skilled birth attendant.

Tanzania was off track for reducing the number of maternal deaths, even with the supports to train midwives and to train non-specialists to do Caesarean sections. The rate of chronic malnutrition, or stunting of children under five, had been at 40 percent for over twenty-five years. Clearly, even with improvements in the mortality rate of children under five, the persistence of chronic malnutrition highlights this important area of concern with Canada's Muskoka Initiative funding. In the Demographic and Health Survey (2010), 46 percent of boys under five and 36 percent of girls were chronically malnourished. This has been largely unchanged since 1991.[4]

From 2004 to 2010, the use of modern contraception increased from 20 to 27 percent. Building on this nascent momentum for family planning will be important, as the maternal mortality rate cannot decline without a reduction in the fertility rate (numbers of births per woman). When only 50 percent of pregnant women have had a skilled birth attendant, improvements in safe delivery are not enough to help reduce the number of women who die in labour and delivery. This is why family planning, which reduces high risk births and prevents abortion, is an important strategy to save the lives of pregnant women.

In addition, deaths of children under five are much fewer if babies are spaced four years apart compared to two years apart (74:136 deaths per 1,000 births). Use of contraception is higher in women who are educated: 22 percent of women with no education space their births compared with 52 percent for women with secondary education or more. Any strategy to help women learn to read, including as adults through non-formal education, would complement the strong government priority for universal primary education in terms of improving the demand-side (women requesting enhanced health services) for the uptake of maternal, neonatal, and child health (MNCH) services, including family planning. There were many missed opportunities for birth spacing: half the women who were non-users of contraception had visited a health facility in the previous year, but one-third of these did not discuss family planning. While the modern contraceptive prevalence rate rose from 7 percent in 1991 to 27 percent in 2010 (from 2005–2010 on the basis of uptake in rural women), the unmet need (women who want to space births but are not doing so) was not reduced, according to the 2010 Tanzania Demographic and Health Survey. Still, 17 percent of teenagers became pregnant, and these are higher risk births. The support Canada has given to family planning in this context through various strategies is, therefore, extremely important as a strategy to reduce the numbers of deaths of pregnant women, newborns and children under five.

Although illegal in Tanzania, intimate partner violence was experienced by one-third of women in the previous twelve months.[5] There are geographic variations: only 10 percent of women in Zanzibar have been beaten. Overall, in Tanzania, 10 percent of women aged 15–49 were forced into their first act of coitus, and overall 20 percent of women of reproductive age have experienced sexual violence. Nearly 10 percent of women have experienced physical violence during pregnancy. Fifteen percent of women in Tanzania have been subjected to FGC (female genital cutting), with wide regional ethnic variations and socio-cultural variations (incidence decreases as women's education and wealth increases), according to the 2010 Tanzania Demographic and Health Survey. This could potentially change: 90 percent of men and women think the practice should be discontinued.

There now needs to be a more concerted effort on the three main drivers of maternal and neonatal mortality: birth spacing, skilled attendants at delivery, emergency obstetric care, and managing inequities in care. How have development partners such as Canada contributed to this challenge? In Tanzania funding had been provided to United Nations agencies, non-governmental organizations, and the Tanzanian government. The Canadian government's Department of Foreign Affairs, Trade and Development has funded civil society organizations in the poorer Lake and Western Zones. We helped improve the distribution of workers and training for task shifting, so non-specialists can do emergency obstetric care. We helped improve the distribution of drugs and technology innovations using eHealth. Projects were well-linked with regional and community health management teams, and quality of services improved. Strong community participation also helped make projects more sustainable. New services such as four comprehensive emergency obstetric care sites were added, and research documented the importance of the role of the community health worker to bridge systems. Equity was addressed by prioritizing underserved areas, but, still, Tanzania needs to address incentives to bring midwives to underserved areas.[6]

Canada has become a lead development partner in health in Tanzania. Health systems strengthening included innovations such as tracking near misses — women and newborns who had nearly died – in order to prevent future recurrences. Still, many facilities lack water, so delivering women have to buy and bring their own water for deliveries, adding to their costs. Remaining problems are the lack of medicines such as misoprostol for post-partum hemorrhage, an innovation that Canada helped fund in South

Sudan but which is not yet allowed in Tanzania because of concerns about "repurposing" this medication to cause abortions.

I was happy to be back in Tanzania. Two old friends, Sheila Robinson, who I had worked with in Nepal, and Susan Smith, who I worked with on a variety of assignments, were here on an additional but related assignment. We tried to coordinate our work. As we prepared for meetings, as we visited projects in the field, I would be at times in my hotel in Dar es Salaam in the evening. On five different occasions, as I got ready for bed in the middle of the night, my computer called out to me. I had stored Jens Hasfeldt's dying message to me. He was the one who sent me to Tanzania for the preparation of that first health sector-wide approach. And he died, many years later, when I was on assignment in his stead, in Papua New Guinea. Unprompted, his voice called out from my computer, "Gretchen? I am wishing you well on this work. It is important. Call me when you can."

Even I know that I can no longer call my deceased friend Jens. But he would be thrilled to know the gap in coverage of mother-and-child health services between rich and poor people is narrowing; 40 percent of poor women get family planning compared to 70 percent of wealthy women; over 80 percent of women of all income groups get at least one prenatal visit; and 40 percent of poor women and 60 percent of wealthy women get four or more antenatal visits. Three times more wealthy women get a skilled birth attendant (30:90), showing the difficulty improving maternal health compared with child health. Immunization of infants, Vitamin A distribution, and treatment of diarrhea also shows inequities and gaps in coverage by income quintile but not as severe as treatment for pneumonia, which is more expensive both to seek care and also to get antibiotics. Government is seeing these differentials, including regional differences showing more needs in the Lake and Western Zones, which will now get priority attention.[7]

Bhutan, 2016

I had forgotten how far away, measured in miles or mindsets, Bhutan is. I had last been there in 2001. There was now a direct flight from Toronto to Delhi, but hotel rooms in the Delhi airport that, of course, were nearly impossible to check into (several hours of negotiating to be allowed into a prepaid room, which I discovered had no water), and the usual complicated connection to Druk Air. And then drifting and spiraling down into Paro Airport.

I found myself so happy to see men in the traditional *goh* dress. It was such an expansive feeling to be in a country with a high level of organization, with speakers arriving from different countries, complex schedules of planes to be met, and some coming overland through India. The conference organizers were not sure about the visas for some delegates. Delegates were already en route from China; visas hopefully would be available when they arrived. My own had taken several misfires before being granted.

The winding road from Paro to Thimphu felt so resonant, but as we approached Thimphu, I saw so many more cars, so many more buildings, so many more Indian labourers toiling on the roadworks!

Nancy, a long-time Canadian friend living in Bhutan had suggested I present a paper on mother-and-child health at a conference to be held in Thimphu in November, 2016. I had always seen Bhutan as a success story and was excited to develop my thoughts for the paper. I wanted to look not only at their outstanding achievements, but also at what was left to do. And since many countries would have to face the same challenges, how could an analysis of Bhutan's experience develop strategies that could help not only themselves but also others?

Many countries have reached the goals of reducing the number of deaths of infants and children under five. Fewer countries have improved the health of pregnant women. But globally the maternal mortality ratio almost halved between 1990 and 2013, from 380 to 210 maternal deaths per 100,000 live births. In Bhutan the maternal mortality ratio was a success story. Its maternal mortality ratio was 120 deaths of pregnant women per 100,000 live births, against a much higher regional average of 190. The maternal mortality ratio also fell way below its own target of 225. In 1990 Bhutan eliminated newborn and maternal tetanus through immunization and increased access to emergency obstetric care to 12 percent (the World Health Organization estimates 5–15 percent of pregnant women will need this help). It also increased access to a skilled birth attendant (midwife or doctor) fourfold, from 15 percent of pregnant women having a skilled birth attendant in 1994 to 64.5 percent in 2010. This resulted from an increase in the number of doctors and nurses, from 50 and 335 respectively in 2002 to 244 doctors and 957 nurses in 2014. But still, 90 percent of urban women have a skilled birth attendant compared to 54 percent of rural women, and 95 percent of rich women have a skilled birth attendant compared to 34 percent of poor women, almost a threefold difference.[8]

So to improve mother-and-child health, there needs to be a mix of "supply side," or trained, health workers in the right geographic areas. Bhutan also worked on the "demand side" (reducing poverty, educating and empowering women, etc.) which has been shown to increase the use of health services. In 2007–12, poverty levels decreased from 23 percent to 12 percent. Gender parity has been achieved in primary and secondary education. Family planning, which is the most cost-effective intervention to improve maternal, newborn, and child health outcomes, has been very successful, with a fertility rate decline to 2.3 children per woman of reproductive age and a contraceptive prevalence rate at 66 percent.[9]

───────◆───────

I am so happy to be here. My breathing is getting deeper. I enjoy being cozy at Nancy's home, with its Bhutanese woven cushions, sense of serenity, and my calm awareness of her decades of faithfulness to Canadian support for education in Bhutan. One night we go for dinner with a couple, Grant and Dort, who met in Bhutan as volunteer teachers years ago and are here to celebrate their twenty-fifth anniversary. We share a meal in a small restaurant we all remember from previous times. Nancy is the experienced one — she has been here for decades. An autographed photo from the former King for her birthday graces her walls. Grant and Dort had lived here for years and had married and had children, and their lives changed because of Bhutan. And me? A few visits of several weeks each over a decade, helping to design two successive five-year health plans, I feel honoured to be close enough, to be trusted, in one of the most remarkable countries I have been privileged to work in.

The conference is in the daytime. After hours, Grant and Dort and I take a drive to see the new Buddha near Thimphu. Vajrayana Buddhism is the state religion of Bhutan and is derived from Tibetan Buddhism. Almost three-quarters of the population of Bhutan are Buddhist, the other one-quarter are Hindu. Some of these Hindu people are in the south where people of Nepali background live, and some are Indians who work in Bhutan.

We proceed slowly up a long, winding fifty-three kilometre drive 328 feet above Thimphu. The Buddha Dordenma is massive: 200 feet tall, made in bronze but gilded in gold. The body with the lotus is 138 feet tall, and the throne beneath the Buddha is 66 feet tall. High on a hill, the Buddha is surrounded by prayerful people, monks in burgundy or saffron robes, beating drums, chanting, walking clockwise. This is a several-day prayer celebration for world peace. Grant, Dort, and I walk clockwise, with the hums of the prayerful walking beside us. The slight smoke of incense, its scent wafts, a drifting haze.

It's timely, to pray for world peace: Americans are about to pick a president, and Nancy and I watch TV in the evening. Political pundits TV said that Hillary Clinton was sure to win. As it turns out, this is not the case, and President Donald Trump is elected. In the morning, on my walk to the university campus, I walk clockwise three times around the temple, go into the sacred temple, and am calmed by the quiet throng of believers with prayer beads. No words, simple, sacred, and then we're on to our days of work.

Some sessions are held in the downtown campus, and we have to be picked up by bus and taken to a larger venue outside the main town. There are other delegates on the bus, some from India, some from China; we chat easily. I have so missed having conversations about larger global health themes. I have so missed speaking with people who are not white Canadians. I had a life of travelling and working with different cultures, in different regions, where I was in the minority as a white, middle-class Canadian. In my work in northern Ontario, Canada, most of my colleagues and patients are white. Our perspective is narrowed to the Ontario context or, on occasion, it broadens to include the American political situation. It is thrilling to speak with colleagues about HIV prevention in India, skilled birth attendants in China, the reduction in maternal mortality in Nepal, and innovations in health worker training in Thailand.

In the sessions, I speak with midwives. We talk about the fact that over half the deaths related to pregnancy in Bhutan are from post-partum hemorrhage. Is this from lack of the medicine misoprostol, which can be given easily in a low-technology setting to prevent deaths from bleeding? Or is this because 50 percent of women are anemic in pregnancy, so even a small bleed can lead to death? I raise the point in the large group session. Only the most senior specialist can order misoprostol. There are fears it can be used illegally to terminate pregnancy. A lively discussion ensues, with the midwives all speaking from their own experiences and requesting greater access to misoprostol and to the senior obstetrician.[10] I am happy to have been part of the debate.

At the closing ceremonies, various dignitaries are on the stage. There are speeches. I catch the eye of one of the senior men on the platform. He is now honoured as *Dasho*. We greet as he leaves the stage. Two successive five-year plans for health had been carefully crafted under his leadership, and with my help. We each smile shyly. I am thrilled to see the progress the country has made. I am honoured with the warm handshake he gives me, recognizing me after fifteen years.

When I go home to my northern Ontario rural medicine practice, I assist a colleague, Nicole, with a Caesarean section. She is a family doctor, with extra skills in obstetrics. She is part of the solution to help reduce the inequities of urban and well-off women in Canada that have more access to obstetric care than rural women. I wish Bhutan could see that not only obstetricians and gynecologists do this work. She agrees that misoprostol can complement oxytocin for management of hemorrhage. I send an email to Bhutan, excited to still be in conversation with such a success story. I also explain that even in Canada, there are huge differences in obstetric care between rural and urban areas, and between income levels. In rural areas, there are more induced labours, higher rates of premature deliveries, less availability of obstetricians so family doctors provide emergency obstetric care, and more women who have to leave their home communities to deliver.[11] These are problems we can share, with solutions we can also share.

Ay, ay, ay, ay
Canta y no llores
Porque cantando se allegran
Cielito lindo, los corazones.

Ay, ay, ay, ay
Sing and don't cry
Because by singing,
The sky lightens and gladdens the heart.

— Quirino Mendoza y Cortés, 1882

Acknowledgements

This second edition of *A Doctor's Quest* draws on both my own work since the 2012 edition and changes in the global understanding of the determinants of reproductive, mother, newborn, and child health. I was fortunate to act as the health specialist on the 2015 formative evaluation of Canada's support, $2.85 billion of assistance to improve maternal and child health, launched at the G8/20 Muskoka Summit in 2010. The evaluation included country assessments in South Sudan, Tanzania, and Nigeria as well as reviews of UN programs and NGO projects. Additional assignments in Laos and Bhutan since the first edition contributed complementary perspectives. My writing mentors, Karen Connelly, Isobel Huggan, and John Bemrose, provided continuing encouragement. I am grateful to Dundurn for suggesting this second edition, to the many audiences of faith-based groups, non-governmental organizations (NGOs), libraries, and bookstores, and to the media who publicized the first edition and showed me that people from all walks of life care deeply about how we as a global community can help to catalyze positive change for the world's most vulnerable. I also wish to honour my mother, Helen

Pereira, who wrote five books between the ages of sixty and eighty-three, and who passed away in February 2018.

I should also point out that all the names of patients in *A Doctor's Quest* have been changed. Colleagues have a mix of actual and altered names. On occasion, events that occurred in several assignments have been compressed into one for the purposes of flow and focus.

Appendix 1

A White Mud Letter to a Dear Friend

My face is covered in white mud. Wet and stiff, it was gathered from one special bank on the left-hand side of the road on a stretch three hours from Wabag, in Enga, Papua New Guinea, in sight of a waterfall, high in the grey-green hills before Mount Hagen. To mourn in the Enga Highlands, you smear your face with this clay, which at first seems a dull putty colour but as it dries, and your face tightens and stings slightly, turns quite white.

I am typing alone in my room in Port Moresby. It's midnight, and the white mud on my face is drying. As the tears fall, streaks furrow in the white clay.

Jens, I am mourning you in the Enga way. And I am mourning Papua New Guinea — so loved by you that your dying wish, which couldn't be granted, was one last visit to try to put things right.

I wore my white shell necklace when I made my presentation today. I told Theresa's story and the stories of the unmet promises. The important officials at the National Department of Health and at the United Nations looked at their watches, apologized, and then said they had to go to another meeting.

Jens, twenty years ago we met, full of our own hopes. We made our own promises to fight for change. We had no career ambitions. We would challenge any organization; we would tell it like it was; we would delight in pissing everyone off! We would speak for those who couldn't speak for themselves. We committed to be ruthlessly independent, to not compromise for our own gain but only if it could help the marginal and dispossessed. And we did that. We worked for NGOs and pretty much all the development partners and poor countries in Asia, Sub-Saharan Africa, and the South Pacific.

You have died, and I am living on, but what is our legacy? What have all of us in development achieved with all of this? We can see the progress in education, but still there are large gaps in education between rich and poor, man and woman. We can see the subtle changes in the status of women, but still it is improvements in maternal health that are moving most slowly. We can see the number of deaths of children falling, but newborns continue to die through neglect of their pregnant mothers. This is the work of more than one lifetime. You have had yours, and mine continues, but do we see enough generations to follow us? We have witnessed, but who listens?

I am wailing, silently. I will wash my face and sleep and dream of Theresa's words:

> I am poor.
> I do not have the freedom that you have as a woman. One day my child was playing, the next day he had died. I have no education.
> Why are women dying giving life?
> I am tired of seeing HIV as the price of wealth. Where are our leaders? Why have they forgotten us? We are still waiting.

Outside, the night is a velvet stillness. A full moon rises lazily in a deep, smoky violet sky. As I lie seeking sleep, my hands hold Theresa's shell necklace. I am comforted by her trust in me. I will bring her story and the stories of others I meet on these journeys beyond her own borders.

Appendix 2

Timeline of Missions

Chapter	Country	Missions
1	Uganda	1987–2007: Twelve missions for different development partners (Germany, Denmark, Sweden, Ireland, the World Bank, and the United Nations Population Fund) to strengthen training of primary health-care workers, develop and assess health projects in underserved regions, and evaluate success of national HIV prevention program.
	Sudan	1989: Planning primary health-care project in Darfur and other regions.
	South Sudan	2015: Formative evaluation of Muskoka Maternal, Newborn, and Child Health Initiative.

Chapter	Country	Missions
2	Bangladesh	1990–2009: Twenty-two missions for different development partners, including Canada, Denmark, World Vision, the World Bank, and the United Nations Population Fund, to plan and evaluate maternal and child health and family planning on both project and national levels.
	Nepal	1991–93: Three missions for CIDA to monitor the development of community health and development projects.
	Ghana	1992–96: Seven missions to strengthen maternal and child health in the poorest area of northern Upper West Region;
		2007: Appraisal of Danida's support to the health sector, including HIV/AIDS;
		2008: Two missions with the United Nations Population Fund on strengthening maternal health.
	Global Reflection	2018: Various.
3	Bangladesh	See Chapter 2.
	Ghana	See Chapter 2.
	Ethiopia	1994: Evaluation of the Canadian-funded training of public health physicians.
	Nigeria	2015: Health specialist for evaluation of Muskoka Maternal, Newborn, and Child Health Initiative.

Chapter	Country	Missions
4	China	1996: Planning of a mother-and-child project in Yunnan Province for CIDA. China has committed substantial resources to achieve universal education.
	Botswana	1998: For UNICEF and on behalf of the UN Theme Group to develop a national adolescent sexual and reproductive health strategy. 2006: Team leader funded by the World Bank, of the inception mission of the Mid-Term Review of the National AIDS Control Program.
	Uganda	See Chapter 1.
	Afghanistan and Nigeria	2015: Health specialist for evaluation of the Muskoka Maternal, Newborn, and Child Health Initiative.
5	Indonesia	1998, 1999, 2000: Missions for CIDA, Asian Development Bank, and the World Bank to support provincial maternal health care and family planning.
	Zimbabwe	1999: In a two-member team to plan a large program for the entire health sector funded by the Danish and other European governments.
	Bhutan	1996–2001: Six missions for Danida to help develop the health sector strategy for one decade and to evaluate human resource training.
	Bangladesh	See Chapter 2.

Chapter	Country	Missions
	Zambia	1992–2001: Six missions to review family planning and urban primary health care and plan support to the whole health sector, including maternal and reproductive health, for the government of Zambia and different development partners.
	Tanzania	1999–2006: Ten missions for different development partners, including CIDA, Denmark, and the World Bank, to strengthen HIV prevention, reproductive health, and primary health care and assess the entire health sector, including the plateau in maternal health.
	Papua New Guinea	2006–9: Six missions to independently monitor and review progress and constraints in the whole health sector on behalf of the governments of Papua New Guinea, Australia, and New Zealand, as well as the United Nations.
6	Tanzania	See Chapter 5.
	Papua New Guinea	See Chapter 5.
7	Malawi	1990: Two missions, one to plan a district primary health-care project (German government) and one to evaluate training of orthopedic clinical officers (Canada).
	Papua New Guinea	See Chapter 5.
	Ghana, Global	See Chapter 2.

Chapter	Country	Missions
8	Bangladesh	2009–10: Co-team leader of the mid-term evaluation of the Campaign to End Fistula (United Nations Population Fund).
	Laos	2012: Health specialist for Luxemburg Development mid-term evaluation.
	Nigeria	2015: Health specialist for evaluation of the Muskoka Maternal, Newborn, and Child Health Initiative.
Endings	Papua New Guinea	See Chapter 5.
	Tanzania Global	2015: Evaluation of Muskoka Maternal, Newborn, and Child Health Initiative.
	Bhutan	2016: Presenter at Mother and Child Health Conference.

Appendix 3

Coda — Where Are We Now?

Countdown to 2030[1] looks at mother, newborn, and child survival across a continuum of reproductive care as part of the tracking of progress towards the Sustainable Development Goals.[2] Countries with the largest problems are closely tracked. So, for example, China, discussed in the book, does not represent a country with high death rates of pregnant women and children under five, so it is not analyzed in the Countdown to 2030, but Nigeria is because of risk factors and a large population in which the largest number of women die in pregnancy of any country in the world. Each country is granted a composite coverage index assessing how well the basic interventions across the continuum of reproductive health care are addressed by each country.[3]

Following the chapters in the book, this is how progress is being tracked according to these following important determinants of health by the Countdown to 2030.

I Am Poor

The Countdown looks at equity, comparing the top and bottom income quintiles in terms of access and utilization of basic health services for adolescents, women of child-bearing age, newborns, and children under five: family planning with modern methods; four antenatal visits, which is the recommended minimum according to the World Health Organization; neonatal tetanus protection; skilled birth attendants; postnatal care for mother and newborn; breastfeeding; immunization; and care seeking for pneumonia and diarrhea. The population living below the international poverty line (US$1.90 a day) is also tracked.

I Do Not Have the Freedom That You Have as a Woman

The indicator tracking the percentage of women who have completed secondary education is a good proxy indicator on the status of women. There are other indicators tracked elsewhere in global documents, for example, looking at the percentage of women in public office. The Demographic and Health Surveys done in many countries look at issues such as teenaged pregnancy, violence against women, or female genital mutilation as indicators on gender. In most of the countries examined in this book, more women than men think violence against women is acceptable (for burning the food, having dinner late, disagreeing with your husband, going out without permission, etc.). This shows it is with women that the seeds of change have to be sown. Goal 5 of the Sustainable Development Goals, to achieve gender equality and empower all women and girls, will help countries keep this important focus.

One Day My Child Was Playing, the Next Day He Had Died

In Countdown to 2030, trends in neonatal and children-under-five deaths are tracked: causes of death of children under five; stillbirth rate; percentage of deaths under five that are of newborns (i.e., reflecting the need for improved delivery care); coverage of interventions to improve child health such as breastfeeding, immunization, Vitamin A distribution, and treatment of pneumonia and diarrhea; and nutritional status assessing both wasting (acute) and stunting (chronic).

I Have No Education

The percentage of women who have completed secondary education is tracked. Women with secondary education have better utilization of maternal and child health care and family planning services, and have lower maternal and child death rates.

Why Are Women Dying Giving Life?

Antenatal care, the percentage of women delivering with a skilled birth attendant, access to emergency obstetric care, postnatal care, maternal deaths and their causes, met need for use of modern contraception, teenaged pregnancy, anemia and, whether women are given iron and folic acid supplements are all closely analyzed.

I Am Tired of Seeing HIV as the Price of Wealth

The percentage of pregnant women living with HIV who receive anti-retroviral drugs is listed; for example, in Uganda, the epicentre of the epidemic, more than 95 percent of pregnant women with HIV receive this therapy. Similarly, in Botswana, where the HIV prevalence rate is the second or third worst in the world, after Swaziland, and as of 2017, after Lesotho, 94 percent of pregnant women receive anti-retrovirals.

Where Are Our leaders? Why Have They Forgotten Us?

Government policies and plans to promote mother-and-child health as follows:

- provide access to family planning for teenagers without parental or spousal consent (teenaged pregnancy and abortion are major causes of maternal deaths)
- provide access to safe legal abortion
- policies to protect pregnant women
- follow international code on limiting breastmilk substitutes
- fortify basic foods such as wheat, maize, and rice
- have costed plans to implement maternal, newborn, and child health strategies
- involve civil society in national planning and review processes
- track maternal deaths
- follow government expenditures on health and, more specifically,

on reproductive, adolescent, maternal, newborn, and child health
- have available life-saving commodities for maternal, newborn, and child health
- have emergency obstetric care facilities, the appropriate numbers of health workers, and midwives authorized for specific life-saving tasks.

The following table shows the composite coverage index for a wide range of interventions across the continuum of reproductive, maternal, newborn, child, and adolescent health care for countries discussed in the book. Details can be accessed at Countdown2030.org.

COVERAGE ACROSS REPRODUCTIVE, MATERNAL, NEWBORN, CHILD, AND ADOLESCENT HEALTH	
Countdown to 2030 Composite Coverage Index	Country
49%	Afghanistan
65% (skilled birth attendance has doubled since 2006)	Bangladesh
Not ranked but steadily declining deaths of pregnant women, newborns, and children under five.	Bhutan
Not ranked (no equity, diarrhea or pneumonia treatment, or postnatal care data available, but numbers of maternal and under-five deaths falling, neonatal deaths plateauing).	Botswana
Not a country with a large number of deaths in pregnant women or children under five so not tracked.	China
35%	Ethiopia
65%	Ghana
75%	Indonesia
55%	Laos
77%	Malawi
66%	Nepal

Countdown to 2030 Composite Coverage Index	Country
38% (marked regional inequity)	Nigeria
Unranked; no data on equity or on adolescent health; 50% have a skilled birth attendant.	Papua New Guinea
Not ranked; 41% of rich women have a skilled birth attendant compared to 8% of poor women; 4% of women have completed secondary education.	South Sudan
52% (wide regional disparity)	Sudan
58%	Uganda
70%	Zambia
73% (treatment of pneumonia dropping and a recent upward trend in maternal deaths)	Zimbabwe

Note: The composite coverage index is used to monitor progress and inequalities in universal health coverage and is based on the average value of separate coverage indicators. The individual indicators are listed under each chapter heading. (Wehrmeister FC, Restrepo-Mendez MC, Franca GVA, Victora CG, and Barros AJD, (2016). Summary indices for monitoring universal coverage in maternal and child health care: Bull World Health Organ 94:903-12. DOI 10.2471/BLT.16.173138 countdown2030.org/countdown-news/summary-index-can-be-used-to-monitor-maternal-and-child-health-care-coverage).

WE ARE STILL WAITING

We are still waiting, but this is a time for cautious optimism. Globally, there have been great improvements in maternal, newborn, and child health. An increased focus on equity, on challenges such as conflict countries (e.g., South Sudan), and on trying to ensure geographic, financial, and cultural barriers to delivery care are removed will take time. The problems of the lack of skilled health workers and the distribution of skilled health workers that favours richer countries and regions need innovative strategies such as task shifting: for example, teaching non-specialist doctors or midwives to do Caesarean sections and providing incentives for health-care providers in underserved regions. Similarly, community-based interventions for childhood illness, in which basic health workers have simple medicines to treat common illnesses including malaria, diarrhea, and pneumonia have been shown to bring low-cost interventions to the poor and reduce death rates of children under five.

NOTES

INTRODUCTION

1. Chelsea Nash, "Maternal, Child Health: Bureaucrats Bolster Liberals' Focus on Family Planning," *Hill Times*, May 18, 2016.
2. Richard Horton, "Offline, Canada's Big Promise," *Lancet*, June 7, 2014.
3. Countdown to 2030 Collaboration, "Countdown to 2030: Tracking Progress Towards Universal Coverage for Reproductive, Maternal, Newborn, and Child Health," *Lancet*, January 30, 2018.
4. Global Affairs Canada, "Formative Evaluation of Canada's Contribution to the Maternal, Newborn and Child Health (MNCH) Initiative," December 2015, international.gc.ca/gac-amc/publications/evaluation/2016/eval_mnch-smne.aspx.
5. Ibid.
6. Countdown to 2030 Collaboration, "Countdown to 2030."

Chapter 1: I Am Poor

1. Ali Mari Tripp, *Museveni's Uganda: Paradoxes of Power in a Hybrid Regime* (Boulder, CO: Lynne Rienner, 2010). Yoweri Kaguta Museveni assumed office a year before, at the end of January 1986, helped to end Idi Amin's harsh dictatorship from 1971 to 1979, and then toppled Milton Obote's 1980–85 regime. He has helped bring down HIV rates and has presided over a period of economic and political stability, though the northern regions of the country remain an ongoing humanitarian emergency conflict. Since assuming power, however, he has become heavily involved in the war in the Democratic Republic of the Congo, which included conflicts over access to diamonds. He has abolished legislation that would have ended his possibility to run again in the 2006 presidential election and has been actively harassing the democratic opposition.

2. Albert Kilian, *HIV/AIDS Control in Kabarole District, Uganda* (Eschborn: GTZ, 2002), hivhealthclearinghouse.unesco.org/sites/default/files/resources/Uganda_GTZ_HIVAIDS_Control_Kabarole_District_Uganda.pdf. The GTZ-funded Basic Health Services Project also increased funding for HIV/AIDS and adolescent health. By 2000 the HIV positivity of teenage pregnant girls had fallen from 30 percent to one-third of the level before the GTZ support. A massive national effort had delivered AIDS prevention messages through schools, churches, mosques, traditional healers, and grassroots organizations. The project we helped design in 1987 in the west was still providing improved primary health care to the people of those regions. GTZ had helped to bridge the condom gap and had targeted adolescents to reduce HIV and also adolescent high-risk pregnancy, which both contributed to maternal deaths.

3. National Bureau of Statistics, *Sudan Household Health Survey* (Sudan: National Bureau of Statistics, 2006), ssnbss.org/sites/default/files/2016-08/Sudan_Household_Health_Survey_Report_2006.pdf; Gretchen Roedde, *Sudan Country Report: Thematic Evaluation of National Programmes and UNFPA Experience in the Campaign to End Fistula* (Rumst, Belgium: hera, 2009). Maternal health has improved

slowly in Sudan. Still, only 2 percent of women have emergency obstetric care, most of them in the top socio-economic quintile (WHO suggests 5 to 15 percent of women will need emergency obstetric care). Only educated, affluent women deliver with a midwife, despite efforts to train more midwives and place them in rural areas. Thousands of women every year still suffer from obstetric fistula. In Darfur the prevalence of fistula is very high because of the lack of facilities to treat emergency obstetric complications in most localities, lack of referral of complicated cases to hospital, low coverage of villages by skilled birth attendance, and ignorance.

4. National Bureau of Statistics, *Sudan Household Health Survey*, 160. More than fifteen years later in 2006 after our work in 1989, one-third of children under five in Sudan were still moderately or severely malnourished and only one-third of children under five were immunized.

5. Countdown to 2015, "South Sudan Health Data — 2014 Profile," *Countdown to 2030*, countdown2030.org/documents/2014Report/ SouthSudan_Country_Profile_2014.pdf. In 2006–7, the Countdown to 2015 estimated an MMR of 1,107 deaths per 100,000 live births. Some estimates are now even higher, at over 2,000 per 100,000 live births, as per the World Bank and WHO. See data.worldbank. org/indicator/SH.STA.MMRT and who.int/gho/maternal_health/ countries/ssd.pdf. One-third of women were married before the age of eighteen. Less than half of all births (49.2 percent) were attended by a qualified health professional.

6. Ibid. Waiting and working for change in Sudan has shown elusive results. A large percentage of the population still lives far from medical facilities. Poverty is widespread — almost 90 percent of the people live on less than one dollar a day. About 40 percent of women have no access to medical care during their pregnancies, and the maternal mortality ratio is very high (the first estimate of 509 maternal deaths out of 100,000 live births has now been estimated between 1,000 and 2,000.) Only 6 percent of women in the south deliver with a trained birth attendant. One of the most extreme forms of female genital cutting, which includes stitching up of the vagina, is

practised widely in the country and is thought to contribute to poor pregnancy outcomes. Our project with GTZ was never implemented, since northern Sudan wouldn't allow support for Darfur.

7. World Bank and WHO estimates are over 2000 in 2015 for Maternal Mortality. See data.worldbank.org/indicator/SH.STA.MMRT and who.int/gho/maternal_health/countries/ssd.pdf.

8. "Fragile States Index 2018," *Fund for Peace*, fundforpeace.org/fsi/data.

9. Olympio Attipoe, Biplove Choudhary, and Nicholas Jonga, *An Analysis of Government Budgets in South Sudan from a Human Development Perspective*, UN Discussion Paper South Sudan, August 2014, ss.undp.org/content/dam/southsudan/library/Discussion%20 Papers/SS-Discussion%20paper%20final.pdf.

10. Kersten Knipp, "SIPRI: Global Military Spending Rose to $1.7 Trillion in 2017," *DW*, May 1, 2018, dw.com/en/sipri-global-military-spending-rose-to-17-trillion-in-2017/a-43610647.

Chapter 2: I Do Not Have the Freedom That You Have as a Woman

1. "Maternal and Neonatal Health in Bangladesh," *UNICEF*, January 2009.

2. WHO in South-East Asia, "Bangladesh and Family Planning: An Overview," WHO, 2003, searo.who.int/entity/child_adolescent/ topics/child_health/fp-ban.pdf.

3. House of Commons International Development Committee, *Maternal Health: Fifth Report of Session 2007–08* (London: House of Commons, 2008), 1:35.

4. Prakash Dev Pant et al., *Investigating Recent Improvements in Maternal Health in Nepal: Further Analysis of the 2006 Nepal Demographic and Health Survey* (Calverton, MD: Macro International, 2008).

5. Ibid.

6. See Appendix 3 Table.

7. Ghana Statistical Service, Noguchi Memorial Institute for Medical Research, and ORC Macro, *Ghana Demographic and Health Survey*

2003 (Calverton, MD: GSS, NMIMR, and ORC Macro, 2004), chapters 5, 8–9.

8. Ibid., 129.

9. Ibid., 146, 150. There is an inverse correlation between women who have a skilled birth attendant and have low status, reflected by the number of reasons a woman thinks wife-beating is justified. Just over 25 percent of women who believe five or more reasons justify wife-beating have a skilled birth attendant in Ghana. Even by 2003, less than one-third of women in Upper West Region had a skilled birth attendant.

10. Immpact, *Implementation of Free Delivery Policy in Ghana* (Legon Accra, Ghana: Immpact, November 2005), mhcghana.com/other/pdf/ Implementation_of_Free_Delivery_Policy_in_Ghana_1.pdf.

11. Sophie Witter et al., "Providing Free Maternal Health Care: Ten Lessons from an Evaluation of the National Delivery Exemption Policy in Ghana," *Global Health Action* 2 (2009).

12. Elizabeth Ardayfio-Schandorf, "Violence Against Women: The Ghanaian Case" (paper presented at UN Division for the Advancement of Women Expert Group Meeting, Geneva, April 11–14, 2005), un.org/womenwatch/daw/egm/vaw-stat-2005/docs/ expert-papers/Ardayfio.pdf.

13. Tony Kusi, Sally Lake, and Gretchen Roedde, *National Consultative Meeting on the Reduction of Maternal Mortality in Ghana: Partnership for Action* (Government of Ghana, November 18, 2011).

14. Ibid.

15. Wikipedia, "Child Sexual Abuse by UN Peacekeepers," last modified July 29, 2018, 00:26, en.wikipedia.org/wiki/Child_sexual_abuse_by_ UN_peacekeepers.

16. Charlotte Alfred, "The Shocking Reality of the Sexual Violence Epidemic in Papua New Guinea," *HuffPost*, March 5, 2016, huffingtonpost.ca/entry/papua-new-guinea-sexual-violence_ us_56d9fca1e4b0ffe6f8e974f2.

17. Jonathan Pearlman, "Why 70 Per Cent of Papua New Guinea's Women Will Be Raped in Their Lifetime," *Telegraph*, February 1, 2016, www.telegraph.co.uk/women/life/why-70-per-cent-of-papua-new-guineas-women-will-be-raped-in-thei.

18. Christopher Albin-Lackey, "Papua New Guinea: Serious Abuses at Barrick Gold Mine," *Human Rights Watch*, February 1, 2011, hrw.org/news/2011/02/01/papua-new-guinea-serious-abuses-barrick-gold-mine.

Chapter 3: One Day My Child Was Playing, the Next Day He Had Died

1. M.K. Munos, C.L. Walker, and R.E. Black, "The Effect of Oral Rehydration Solution and Recommended Home Fluids on Diarrhoea Mortality," *International Journal of Epidemiology* 39 (2010): 75–87.
2. S. Berman, E.A. Simoes, and C. Lanata, "Respiratory Rate and Pneumonia in Infancy," *Archives of Disease in Childhood* 66, no. 1 (1991): 81–84.
3. Gretchen Roedde, Zakir Ahmed, Provat Ch. Barua, et al., *Mid-Term Evaluation of the World Vision Chittagong Child Survival Project* (Bangladesh: World Vision, November 1995).
4. Gretchen Roedde and Kim Streatfield, "Improvements in Health Status" and "Health Service Delivery and Health-Seeking Behavior," background papers for *Bangladesh — Fourth Population and Health Project — End of Project Evaluation* (Dhaka: World Bank, 1999) UNICEF data, accessed at data.unicef.org/country/bgd/.
5. According to UNICEF in 2016, there were further improvements in the male to female ratio (37:32) for the under-five mortality rate. "Bangladesh," UNICEF Data, November 22, 2018, data.unicef.org/country/bgd/.
6. "South Asia Population — Urban Growth: A Challenge and an Opportunity," *World Bank*, UNICEF data, unicef.org/infobycountry/bangladesh_bangladesh_statistics.html.
7. M.J. Uddin et al., "Health Needs and Health-Seeking Behaviour of Street-Dwellers in Dhaka, Bangladesh." *Health Policy and Planning* 24, no. 5 (2009): 385–94. Deaths of street children in Bangladesh rose five times in the fifteen years from 1991. The urban population growth rate in Bangladesh is 6 percent and the national growth rate is 1.15 percent. The infant mortality rate in urban slums in Dhaka

in the late 1990s was nearly double the rate for the rest of the population.

8. Gbenga A. Kayode et al., "Temporal Trends in Childhood Mortality in Ghana: Impacts and Challenges of Health Policies and Programs," *Global Health Action* (2016) doi: 10.3402/gha.v9.31907.

9. Ibid.

10. Disease Control Priorities Project, "Eliminating Malnutrition Could Reduce Poor Countries Disease Burden by One-Third," July 2007, bvsde.paho.org/texcom/nutricion/DCPP-Nutrition.pdf.

11. discap.org/Publications/Conflict%20&%20Conflict%20resolution.pdf.

12. William Faulkner's acceptance speech can be accessed at rjgeib.com/thoughts/faulkner/faulkner.html.

13. Graham Greene's biography can be accessed at greeneland.tripod.com/bio.htm.

14. Ahmed Abdella, "Maternal Mortality Trend in Ethiopia," *Ethiopian Journal of Health Development* 24, no. 1 (2010): 115–22.

15. Ahmed Karadawi, "The Smuggling of the Ethiopian Falasha Through Sudan," *African Affairs* 90, no. 358 (1991): 23–49, jstor.org/pss/722638.

16. *Status Report on Millennium Development Goals 4 and 5 in Africa,* un.org/millenniumgoals/2015_MDG_Report/pdf/MDG%20 2015%20rev%20(July%201).pdf.

17. Gretchen Roedde, Yemane Berhane, and Ato Tsefaye Redda, *End of Project Evaluation: Phase 2 McGill-Ethiopia Community Heath* Project (CIDA, January 20, 1995).

18. Central Statistical Agency [Ethiopia] and MEASURE DHS Project, *Ethiopia Demographic and Health Survey 2011: Preliminary Report* (Addis Ababa, Ethiopia: Central Statistical Agency/Calverton, MD: ICF Macro, September 2011), dhsprogram.com/pubs/pdf/PR10/PR10.pdf.

19. M.A. Travassos et al., "Immunization Coverage Surveys and Linked Biomarker Serosurveys in Three Regions in Ethiopia," *PLoS ONE* 11, no. 3 (2016). Central Statistical Agency [Ethiopia] and ICF, *2016 Ethiopia Demographic and Health Survey Key Findings* (Addis Ababa, Ethiopia: CSA/Rockville, MD: ICF, 2017), dhsprogram.com/pubs/pdf/SR241/SR241.pdf.

20. United Nations Population Fund, *The State of the World's Midwifery Report: Delivering Health, Saving Lives* (New York: UNFPA, 2011), who.int/pmnch/media/membernews/2011/2011_sowmr_en.pdf.

21. Marta Medina and Gretchen Roedde, *Thematic Evaluation of National Programmes and UNFPA Experience in the Campaign to End Fistula,* vol. 2, *Synthesis Report* (Rumst, Belgium: hera, 2010).

22. "Country Profiles: Ethiopia," *UNICEF,* data.unicef.org/country/eth/.

23. Central Statistical Agency and ICF, *2016 Ethiopia Demographic and Health Survey Key Findings* (Addis Ababa, Ethiopia, and Rockville, MD: CSA and ICF, 2017), dhsprogram.com/pubs/pdf/SR241/ SR241.pdf. In the 2016 Demographic and Health Survey, Ethiopia showed continued improvement in under five, neonatal, and infant mortality. Family planning use has increased to one-third of women in union. The median birth interval is almost thirty-six months, which is recommended to improve child survival. There have been improvements of the number of women receiving antenatal care, the quality (tetanus immunization, iron folate tablets, blood pressure taking, and urinalysis) and timing in the pregnancy, and frequency of those visits. Twenty-five percent of births occur in a health facility, which is low, but it was only 5 percent in 2000. There has been an improvement in pregnancy-related mortality.

24. Maternal Health Thematic Fund, *Annual Report 2010* (New York: UNFPA, 2010).

25. Central Statistical Agency and ICEF, *Ethiopia Demographic and Health Survey 2016* (Addis Ababa, Ethiopia, and Rockville, MD: CSA and ICF, 2016), dhsprogram.com/pubs/pdf/FR328/FR328.pdf.

26. Tukur Dahiru, "Surviving the First Day in Nigeria: Risk Factors and Protectors" *American Journal of Public Health Research* 3, no. 4 (2015):128–35.

27. Global Affairs Canada, "Formative Evaluation of Canada's Contribution to the Maternal, Newborn and Child Health (MNCH) Initiative," December 2015, international.gc.ca/gac-amc/publications/ evaluation/2016/eval_mnch-smne.aspx.

Chapter 4: I Have No Education

1. Chinese National Commission for UNESCO and Chinese Adult Education Association, "National Report — Adult Education and Learning in China: Development and Present Situation," July 30, 2008, uil.unesco.org/fileadmin/multimedia/uil/confintea/pdf/ National_Reports/Asia%20-%20Pacific/China.pdf. In China 98.5 percent of counties have "basically eliminated illiteracy among young and middle-aged people" and have "basically popularized nine-year compulsory education."

2. Therese Hesketh, Li Lu, and Zhu Wei Xing, "The Effect of China's One Child Family Policy after 25 Years," *New England Journal of Medicine* 353 (2005): 1171–76.

3. Gretchen Roedde and Yuwa Wong, *Yunnan Ethnic Minorities Maternal and Child Health Care Project — China — Identification Mission* (Horizon Pacific International/CIDA, March 1996).

4. Tom Phillips, "China Ends One-Child Policy After 35 Years" *Guardian*, October 29, 2015, theguardian.com/world/2015/oct/29/ china-abandons-one-child-policy.

5. "Dr. Norman Bethune," *Canadian Medical Hall of Fame*, cdnmedhall. org/inductees/dr-norman-bethune. Norman Bethune was a Canadian physician who worked in both Spain during the Spanish Civil War and in Mao Zedong's China. He was heralded as a hero in China, though it is only more recently that he has become acknowledged in his own country.

6. Health Council of Canada, *Understanding and Improving Aboriginal Maternal and Child Health in Canada* (2011), healthcouncilcanada. ca/files/2.01-HCC_AboriginalHealth_FINAL1.pdf. The infant mortality rate among the Inuit is four times higher and among other Indigenous Peoples two times higher than the general population.

7. N. Edwards and S. Roelofs, "Sustainability: The Elusive Dimension of International Health Projects," *Canadian Journal of Public Health* 97, no. 1 (2006): 45–49. Death rates of pregnant women, infants, and children under five had dropped 30 percent in ten project counties.

8. "Gross National Income Per Capita 2010, Atlas Method and PPP,"

World Development Indicators Database, *World Bank*, July 1, 2011. Botswana purchasing power parity $13,910; China $7,901.

9. "Botswana: Statistics," *UNICEF*, March 2010, unicef.org/ infobycountry/botswana_statistics.html.

10. Working Group of Indigenous Minorities in Southern Africa, "San Literacy."

11. "Incomes Growth in Rural Botswana Lifts Thousands out of Poverty and Decreases Inequality," *World Bank*, December 8, 2015, worldbank. org/en/news/press-release/2015/12/08/incomes-growth-in-rural-botswana-lifts-thousands-out-of-poverty-and-decreases-inequality.

12. "World Health Report: Uganda," WHO, who.int/whr/2004/annex/ country/uga. Uganda spends $14 (as of 2001) per capita total expenditure on health.

13. "Botswana," *WHO*, who.int/countries/bwa. Total expenditure on health per capital (2009): $1,341.

14. "HIV and AIDS in Botswana" *Avert*, September 28, 2018, avert.org/ professionals/hiv-around-world/sub-saharan-africa/botswana.

15. Centre for Health and Gender Equity, "The Case for Comprehensive: Botswana," May 2009, genderhealth.org/files/uploads/change/ publications/botswanacasestudy.pdf.

16. UNAIDS, "Chapter 2: Epidemic Update," *Global Report: UNAIDS Report on the Global AIDS Epidemic, 2010* (WHO, 2010), unaids.org/ globalreport/documents/20101123_GlobalReport_full_en.pdf. It has dropped from second to third place, and its rate of HIV prevalence is now at 23 percent, according to a 2017 UNAIDS report.

17. UNAIDS, "Epidemiological Fact Sheets on HIV/AIDS and Sexually Transmitted Infections, 2004 Update: Botswana," 14.

18. Ibid., 3. The life expectancy had fallen to forty years. In 2005 it fell to 35, but has increased to 64/68, per WHO. See who.int/ countries/bwa.

19. Center for Health and Gender Equity, "The Case for Comprehensive: Botswana." This remains true unless they can obtain parental consent.

20. In 2006 presiding judge Maruping Dibotelo of the High Court of Botswana declared that the government of Botswana had acted

illegally: "The applicants were denied of such possessions (of land in the Central Kalahari Game Reserve) forcibly or wrongly and without their consent." Quote by Judge Maruping Dibotelo in "Botswana Bushmen Win Land Ruling," *BBC News*, December 13, 2006, news.bbc.co.uk/2/hi/africa/6174709.stm. In 2007 human rights groups, including the Botswana Council of Churches, criticized the government of Botswana for delaying the return of the San to their ancestral lands in the Central Kalahari and for the government's refusal to restore health and education services to the Bushmen. They then won the right to return as noted in 2013. See sbs.com.au/news/bushmen-win-right-to-return.

21. Rachelle Winkle Wagner, "An Endless Desert Walk: Perspectives of Education from the San in Botswana, Log No: 04/086," *International Journal of Educational Development* 26, no. 1 (2006): 9.

22. Nathan Chelimo, "Classes Under the Trees: Transitions in Pastoral Communities in Uganda," in *Early Childhood Matters* 107 (Bernard van Leer Foundation, 2006), 36–37, portal.oas.org/Portals/7/Educacion_Cultura/ECD%20Matters%20%20%20%20Transitions%20Van%20leer%20Foundation.pdf. This is now improving with the advent of non-formal education.

23. OCHA, "Uganda," unocha.org/southern-and-eastern-africa-rosea/uganda.

24. "Delivering as One to Kick HIV/AIDS Out of Karamoja," November 29, 2016, reachahand.org/story/delivering-as-one-to-kick-hivaids-out-of-karamoja. UNICEF data, 2014 HIV stats: data.unicef.org/resources/state-worlds-children-2016-statistical-tables/. According to UNICEF, the HIV prevalence nationally was 7.3 percent as of 2014, and Karamoja had increased to 5.6 percent in 2006.

25. Evelyn Kiapi Matsamura, "Renewed War Against Teenage Pregnancies," *IPS*, February 23, 2004, ipsnews.net/2004/02/health-uganda-renewed-war-against-teenage-pregnancies.

26. Sam Okuonzi and Helen Epstein, "Pragmatic Safe Sex, Not Abstinence or Faithfulness, Was Key in Uganda's HIV Decline," *Health Policy and Development Journal* 3, no. 1 (2005): ii–iii.

27. "Adolescent Development," *UNICEF*, unicef.org/uganda/Adol_Dev_print(1).pdf.

28. Uganda Bureau of Statistics (UBOS), Uganda Demographic and Health Survey 2016/2017, ubos.org/onlinefiles/uploads/ubos/ pdf%20documents/2017_UNHS_26092017-Final_Presentation. pdf; Uganda Bureau of Statistics (UBOS) and Macro International, Uganda Demographic and Health Survey 2006 (Calverton, MD: UBOS and Macro International, 2007), measuredhs.com/pubs/pdf/ FR194/FR194.pdf.

29. Norad, "A Review of the Alternative Basic Education Program in Karamoja," 2006, norad.no/om-bistand/publikasjon/ngo-evaluations/2009/a-review-of-the-alternative-basic-education-program-in-karamoja.

30. Global Affairs Canada, "Formative Evaluation of Canada's Contribution."

31. "Malala's Story," Malala Fund, malala.org/malalas-story.

32. Hilary Matfess, "Boko Haram Has Kidnapped More Girls. Here's What We Know," *Washington Post*, March 8, 2018, washingtonpost. com/news/monkey-cage/wp/2018/03/08/boko-haram-has-kidnapped-more-girls-heres-what-we-know.

33. Global Affairs Canada, "Formative Evaluation of Canada's Contribution."

34. Countdown to 2030 Collaboration, "Countdown to 2030."

35. "Multiple Indicator Cluster Survey (MICS4) — 2011 Nigeria, Fourth Round," *National Bureau of Statistics — Nigeria*, January 15, 2018, nigerianstat.gov.ng/nada/index.php/catalog/35.

36. National Bureau of Statistics and UNICEF, *2017 Multiple Indicator Cluster Survey 2016–17, Survey Findings Report*, (Abuja, Nigeria: National Bureau of Statistics and UNICEF, 2017), unicef.org/nigeria/ NG_publications_mics_201617feb2018.pdf.

37. Nuzulack Dausen, "World Bank Re-engages Tanzania on Scrapped Education Plan," Reuters, November 18, 2018, reuters.com/article/ tanzania-worldbank/world-bank-re-engages-tanzania-on-scrapped-education-plan-idUSL8N1XS0J1?feedType=RSS&feedName=rbssFin ancialServicesAndRealEstateNews.

CHAPTER 5: WHY ARE WOMEN DYING GIVING LIFE?

1. Rita Widiadana, "A Matter of Life and Death," *Jakarta Post*, January 13, 2010, thejakartapost.com/news/2010/01/13/a-matter-life-and-death.html.
2. Aid from donors, including UNICEF, have since arranged that the services of the *bidan di desa* are paid for, and they can work in partnership with the traditional birth attendants who are closer to the cultural life of the communities. To help make families more aware of complications in labour and delivery, the United Nations Population Fund has supported episodes such as "Suami Siaga" (Alert Husband) in the local radio drama *Lilin-lilin-di-Depan* (The Guiding Light).
3. Efforts are now underway in Indonesia and globally to have other drugs available such as misoprostol, which can be used to stop post-partum bleeding or bleeding from an incomplete abortion. This can be given rectally and even traditional birth attendants have been trained in its use.
4. Paul Christopher Webster, "Indonesia: The midwife and maternal morality miasma," *Canadian Medical Association Journal*, 185, 2 (February 2013).
5. Jack Corner, "Challenges in achieving MDG 5 target in Indonesia," *dr7ack corner* (blog), January 29, 2011, ridwangustiana.wordpress.com/2011/01/29/indonesia-challenges-to-achieve-mdg-5.
6. The maternal mortality ratio increased from 1990 to 2005 from 440 to 629 per 100,000 live births, but have now decreased back to the 1990 levels according to UNICEF and WHO in 2015. Per UNICEF and WHO: 440 in 1990, 449 in 1995, 590 in 2000, 629 in 2005, 446 in 2010, and 443 in 2015. WHO, "Maternal Mortality in 1990–2015 — Zimbabwe," who.int/gho/maternal_health/countries/zwe.pdf; UNICEF, "Maternal and Newborn Health Disparities in Zimbabwe," data.unicef.org/wp-content/uploads/country_profiles/Zimbabwe/country%20profile_ZWE.pdf.
7. National AIDS Council and Ministry of Health and Child Care, *Global Aids Response Progress Report 2018*, 2017, unaids.org/sites/default/files/country/documents/ZWE_2018_countryreport.pdf.

8. Justin Pearce, "Mugabe's costly Congo venture," *BBC News*, July 25, 2000, news.bbc.co.uk/2/hi/africa/611898.stm.

9. World Bank, *Reproductive Health at a Glance: Zimbabwe*, (World Bank, May 2011), siteresources.worldbank.org/INTPRH/Resources/376374-1282255445143/Zimbabwe52411web.pdf. "Deaths of pregnant women." This remains a continuing, worsening situation. "Zimbabwe has not made progress over the past two decades on maternal health and is not yet on track to achieve its 2015 targets" (p. 1). The Maternal Mortality Ratio in 1990 was 390 per 100,000 live births; as of 2000, it was 670; as of 2008, it was 790 (p. 1, Figure 1).

10. Ibid. "Home deliveries increased nationally ..."

11. "Global Health" USAID, last updated June 4, 2018, usaid.gov/zimbabwe/global-health.

12. "About Bhutan," UNDP, bt.undp.org/content/bhutan/en/home/countryinfo/.

13. Ibid. Women receiving skilled birth attendance doubled between 2000 and 2007.

14. In the 1960s a Canadian Jesuit of Irish Catholic descent, Father William Mackey, met the prime minster of Bhutan, Jigmie Dorji, and his sister, Ashi Tashi, while teaching elite Bhutanese at St. Robert's High School, in Darjeeling, India. An excellent but controversial educator, he was expelled from India during a politically chaotic time and was invited to Bhutan in 1963 by King Jigme Dorji Wangchuck and his brother-in-law, the prime minister, to help establish schools there. Ashi Tashi asked him to concentrate on the east in Tashigang ("auspicious mountain"), which was poor, well populated, and underdeveloped, where she had helped administer a large district. He was to remain in Bhutan until his death in 1995, the year before I first arrived in Bhutan, laying the foundation for modern education in the country. Everyone I met, Bhutanese or expatriate, remembered him with love and respect, and he was honoured at his death by both Jesuits and Buddhists, one of only two foreigners who was named a Son of Bhutan. Thanks to his involvement, Canadian volunteer teachers have continued to come to Bhutan for decades.

15. World Health Organization, *Monitoring Emergency Obstetric Care — A Handbook*, (Geneva, Switzerland: World Health Organization, 2009) 14–15, apps.who.int/iris/bitstream/handle/10665/44121/ 9789241547734_eng.pdf.

16. Howard Solverson, *The Jesuit and the Dragon* (Montreal, QC: Robert Davies Publishing, 1995).

17. Malay Kanti Mridha, Iqbal Anwar, and Marge Koblinsky, "Public Sector Maternal Health Care and Services for Rural Bangladesh," *Journal of Health Population and Nutrition* 27, no. 2 (April 2009): 124–38.

18. USAID and Measure Evaluation, Bangladesh Maternal Mortality and Health Care, *Survey 2016* (2017), measureevaluation.org/resources/ publications/fs-17-245-en/.

19. Chris Simms, "Health Reformers' Response to Zambia's Child Mortality Crisis," (Institute of Development Studies Working Paper 121, 2000), ids.ac.uk/files/Wp121.pdf; and Ron Labonte, Ted Schrecker, and Amit Sen Gupta, *Health for Some: Death, Disease and Disparity in a Globalizing Era* (Toronto, ON: Centre for Social Justice, 2005): 28–32.

20. hera Belgium, *Zambia National Health Strategic Plan 2011–2015 — Joint Health Pre-Appraisal Mission* (Belgium: hera, May 2001); and Euro Health Group, *Health Sector Programme Support Formulation Report for HSPS III* (Danish Ministry of Foreign Affairs and Ministry of Health Zambia, January 2002).

21. Transparency International, *Global Corruption Report 2008: Corruption in the Water Section*, June 25, 2008, 154–55.

22. "Zambia: Health Funding Frozen After Corruption Alleged," IRIN Plus News, May 27, 2009.

23. Dambisa Moyo, *Dead Aid: Why Aid Is Not Working and How There is a Better Way for Africa*, (New York: Farrar, Straus and Giroux, 2009).

24. Central Statistical Office, Ministry of Health, Tropical Diseases Research Centre, University of Zambia, and Macro International, *Zambia: Demographic and Health Survey 2007* (Calverton, MD: Central Statistical Office and Macro International, 2009), dhsprogram.com/ pubs/pdf/FR211/FR211[revised-05-12-2009].pdf.

25. Central Statistical Office, *Zambia: Demographic Health Survey, 2013–14*, March 2015, dhsprogram.com/pubs/pdf/FR304/FR304.pdf.

26. Central Statistical Office, Ministry of Health, Tropical Diseases Research Centre, University of Zambia, and Macro International, *Zambia: Demographic and Health Survey 2007*.

27. "One percent of them had access to a Caesarean section ..." National Bureau of Statistics [Tanzania] and ORC Marco, *Tanzania Demographic and Health Survey 2004–5*, (Dar es Salaam, Tanzania: National Bureau of Statistics and ORC Macro, December 2005), Chapter 9. The poor have much lower rates of skilled birth attendance and emergency obstetric care than the rich as well as less comprehensive antenatal care (i.e., not being told of possible complications or having blood pressure taken, et cetera). Overall the country has a higher C-section rate (3.2 percent), but there are great regional and socio-economic variations. See World Health Organization, "United Republic of Tanzania Country Profile," *Department of Making Pregnancy Safer, 2004* (Geneva, Switzerland: World Health Organization, 2004), 4, who.int/maternal_child_adolescent/events/2008/mdg5/countries/final_cp_tanzania_19_09_08.pdf.

28. "Over 60 percent of women in Tanzania ..." and "Gender inequality index and related indicators," *Human Development Report, 2011*, UNDP, 141, Table 4, hdr.undp.org/sites/default/files/reports/271/hdr_2011_en_complete.pdf.

29. Paul Smithson, with Ifakara Centre for Health Research and Development, *Fair's Fair: Health Inequalities and Equity in Tanzania* (Dar es Salaam, Tanzania: Women's Dignity Project, 2006).

30. The maternal mortality ratio had increased from 529 to 578 per 100,000 live births according to the 2004 Demographic and Health Survey; skilled attendance at delivery had dropped from 50 percent to 47 percent, and the total fertility rate had plateaued at 5.7 births per woman. Since then there have been improvements. The new DHS came out in 2015. National Bureau of Statistics [Tanzania] and ICF, *Tanzania Demographic and Health Survey and Malaria Indicator Survey 2015–16* (Dar es Salaam, Tanzania: National Bureau of Statistics, Rockville, Maryland: ICF, 2016) The updated maternal mortality ratio was 200 per 100,000 live births (p. 323); skilled attendance at delivery was 64 percent (p. 167); and fertility rate was 5.2 births per woman (p. 105).

31. Gretchen Roedde et al., *Technical Review 2006 District Health Services in Tanzania* (Belgium: hera, 2006).

32. National Department of Health [NDoH], PNG, *Ministerial Task Force on Maternal Health in Papua New Guinea* (Port Moresby, PNG: NDoH, May 2009).

33. Independent Monitoring and Review Group, *IMRG Reports 2006– 2009* (Papua New Guinea: November 2006, May 2007, November 2007, June 2008, October 2008).

34. Sinclair Dinnen, "Big Men, Small Men and Invisible Women," *Australian and New Zealand Journal of Criminology* 44, no. 3, December 2011. Nearly 40 percent of the population lived below the poverty line. Assessment of Development Results: Evaluation of UNDP Contribution Papua New Guinea (USA: UNDP, 2011), undp.org/content/dam/undp/library/corporate/Evaluation/Assesment%20of%20development%20results/Papua_New_Guinea/ADR-PNG-2011.pdf. Alison Anis, "Studies link sexual abuse, marital rapes to HIV rise," The National, August 11, 2010. In her article, Ms. Anis reports that Angela Mandie-filer, gender and social development advisor with AusAID and PNG, said that "Twenty-eight percent of women reported that they were sexually abused as children, while 58 percent experienced physical abuse from their partners (domestic violence) and 45 percent reported sexual abuse by their partners (marital rape)."

35. National Statistical Office, *Papua New Guinea Demographic and Health Survey 2006: National Report* (Port Moresby, PNG: National Statistical Office of Papua New Guinea, 2009); see also Australian Government Office of Development Effectiveness, "Executive Summary," *Working Paper No. 1 PNG Country Report. Evaluation of Australian Aid to the Health Sector* (Canberra: Australian Agency for International Development, June 2009), dfat.gov.au/aid/how-we-measure-performance/ode/Documents/working-paper-1-png-country-report.pdf.

36. National Statistical Office, *Demographic and Health Survey* (Port Moresby, PNG: National Statistical Office, 2006).

37. Mick Foster et al., *Working Paper No. 1 PNG Country Report. Evaluation of Australian Aid to the Health Sector* (AusAID Government

Office of Development Effectiveness: 2009), executive summary, dfat.gov.au/aid/how-we-measure-performance/ode/Documents/working-paper-1-png-country-report.pdf.

38. Alison Moores et al., "Education, employment and practice: Midwifery graduates in Papua New Guinea," *Midwifery* (2016), sciencedirect. com/science/article/pii/S0266613816301152.

39. Brian Cross, "The Bougainville Civil War and Fight for Independence" *South Pacific History* (Suite 101), June 8, 2010.

40. "Bougainville promises legal challenge over PNG funding," Radio New Zealand, March 21, 2017, radionz.co.nz/international/pacific-news/327116/bougainville-promises-legal-challenge-over-png-funding.

CHAPTER 6: I AM TIRED OF SEEING HIV AS THE PRICE OF WEALTH

1. For a comprehensive understanding of the interaction between foreign aid and HIV, see the following: Miriam Rabkin et al., "The Impact of HIV Scale-Up on Health Systems: A Priority Research Agenda," *Journal of Acquired Immune Deficiency Syndromes* 52 (November 2009): S6–11; Paula O'Brien and Lawrence O. Gostin, "Health Worker Shortages and Inequalities: The Reform of United States Policy," *Global Health Governance*, vol. 2 (Fall 2008–Spring 2009); Bernard Liese and Gilles Dussault, "The State of the Health Workforce in Sub-Saharan Africa: Evidence of Crisis and Analysis of Contributing Factors" (African Region Human Development working paper series, Washington, DC, World Bank, 2004); See United Nations Population Fund [UNFPA], *The State of the World's Midwifery Report: Delivering Health, Saving Lives* (New York: UNFPA, 2014), for several country reports on Tanzania, including efforts to prioritize midwives in rural areas with incentives, some supported by the Canadian government. Accessed at unfpa.org/sowmy/resources/en/library.htm#country; United States Agency for International Development [USAID], *The Health Sector Human*

Resource Crisis in Africa: An Issues Paper (Washington, DC: Support for Analysis and Research in Africa, 2003), hrhresourcecenter.org/node/33.html.

2. UNFPA, *The National Roadmap Strategic Plan to Accelerate Reduction of Maternal, Neonatal and Child Deaths in Tanzania 2008–2015* (April 2008) p. 59, who.int/pmnch/countries/tanzaniamapstrategic.pdf.

3. The United Republic of Tanzania, *Human Resource for Health and Social Welfare Strategic Plan 2014–2019* (Dar es Salaam, Tanzania: Ministry of Health and Social Welfare, 2014).

4. Sigrid Dräger, Gulin Gedik, and Mario R. Dal Poz, "Health Workforce Issues and the Global Fund to Fight AIDS, Tuberculosis and Malaria: An Analytic Review," *Human Resources for Health* 4 (2006): 23.

5. Pablo Gottret and George Schieber, *Health Financing Revisited: A Practitioner's Guide* (Washington, DC: World Bank, 2006), 131–32.

6. Smithson, *Fair's Fair: Health Inequalities and Equity in Tanzania, Dar es Salaam: Women's Dignity Project, 2006.*

7. Mick Foster and H. Mwinyimvua, "Funding for HIV and AIDS in Tanzania (Public Expenditure Review HIV/AIDS Multisectoral Update for 2004," Ifakara Health Institute, last modified January 14, 2013, ihi.eprints.org/617/.

8. Gretchen Roedde, "Progress and Pain on the Path of Humanitarian Medicine," review of *Globalization and Health: Pathways, Evidence and Policy,* by Ronald Labonté et al., eds., *Canadian Medical Association Journal* 182, no. 12, September 7, 2010.

9. Doris Chou et al., *Trends in Maternal Mortality 1998–2008* (Geneva, Switzerland: World Health Organization, 2010), whqlibdoc.who.int/publications/2010/9789241500265_eng.pdf.

10. Seth Berkley et al., *World Development Report* 1993: *Investing in Health* (Washington, DC: World Bank Group, 1993), whqlibdoc.who.int/publications/2010/9789241500265_eng.pdf.

11. National Aids Spending Assessment for 2005–2006, files.unaids.org/en/media/unaids/contentassets/dataimport/pub/report/2005/NASA_Tanzania_2005_en.pdf.

12. Congressional Budget Justification, Foreign Assistance — Summary Tables — Fiscal Year 2014, p. 34, state.gov/documents/organization/208292.pdf.

13. "12000 Fewer Children Perish Daily in 2010 than in 1990 — UNICEF, WHO," World Health Organization Media Centre news release, who.int/mediacentre/news/releases/2011/child_mortality_estimates_20110915/en.

14. For more information on annual number of deaths from AIDS, see UNAIDS, *World AIDS Day Report: How to Get to Zero: Faster. Smarter. Better.* (Geneva, Switzerland: Joint United Nations Programme on HIV/AIDS, 2011), unaids.org/en/media/unaids/contentassets/documents/unaidspublication/2011/JC2216_WorldAIDSday_report_2011_en.pdf.

15. "Global Health Initiative," *Foreign Assistance*, foreignassistance.gov/Initiative_GH_2012.aspx?FY=2012.

16. Elisabeth Aahman et al., *World Health Report 2005: Make Every Mother and Child Count* (Geneva, Switzerland: World Health Organization, 2005), who.int/whr/2005/whr2005_en.pdf?ua=1.

17. Toni Johnson, "Global Health Spending Priorities," *Council on Foreign Relations Forum*, October 6, 2008.

18. Jeremy Shiffman and Stephanie Smith, "Generation of Political Priority for Global Health Initiatives: A Framework and Case Study of Maternal Mortality," *Lancet*, 370, no. 9595, October 13, 2007: 1370–79.

19. Roger England, "Are We Spending Too Much on HIV?" *British Medical Journal* 334 (February 2007): 344.

20. Independent Review Group on HIV/AIDS, *Report of September 2008* (2008).

21. Asian Development Bank *Papua New Guinea: HIV/AIDS Prevention and Control in Rural Development Enclaves* (2017), adb.org/sites/default/files/project-documents/39033/39033-022-pcr-en.pdf.

CHAPTER 7: WHERE ARE OUR LEADERS? WHY HAVE THEY FORGOTTEN US?

1. Richard Dowden, "Obituary: Dr. Hastings Banda," *Independent*, November 27, 1997, independent.co.uk/news/obituaries/obituary-dr-hastings-banda-1296534.html.

2. UNICEF Factsheet on Malawi. Accessed at unicef.org/infobycountry/malawi_statistics.html.

3. "Malawi's Ex-Dictator, Aides Acquitted of Ordering Four Politicians' Murders," *Los Angeles Times*, December 24, 1995, articles.latimes.com/1995-12-24/news/mn-17461_1_banda.

4. "What Drives Corruption in Malawi and Why It Won't Disappear Soon," *Conversation*, September 20, 2015, theconversation.com/what-drives-corruption-in-malawi-and-why-it-wont-disappear-soon-48183.

5. T. Rosenberg, "Reverse Foreign Aid," *New York Times*, March 25, 2007. "Developing countries as a group are expected to have continued to provide a net transfer of financial resources, of approximately $557 billion, to developed countries in 2010 ... but remained well below the peak of $881 billion in 2007" (69). Source: Rob Vos et al., *World Economic Situation and Prospects 2011*, (New York: United Nations Department of Economic and Social Affairs and United Nations Conference on Trade and Development, 2011) unctad.org/en/Docs/wesp2011_en.pdf.

6. Laura Alfaro, Sebnem Kalemi-Ozcan, and Vadym Volosovych, "Why Doesn't Capital Flow from Rich to Poor Countries? An Empirical Investigation," *Review of Economics and Statistics* 90, no. 2 (November 2005): 347.

7. For more on the lack of nurses, see Ruairí Brugha et al., "Health Workforce Responses to Global Health Initiatives Funding: A Comparison of Malawi and Zambia," *Human Resources for Health* 8 (2010); Ogenna Manafa et al., "Retention of Health Workers in Malawi: Perspectives of Health Workers and District Management," *Human Resources for Health* 7 (2009). An emergency human resources program with donor support has been developed in Malawi in response to the crisis in human resources for health.

8. According to varying estimates, the following countries have deaths rates of pregnant women that exceed one thousand per one hundred thousand live births: Afghanistan, Angola, Central African Republic, Chad, Ethiopia, Guinea-Bissau, Malawi, Mali, Niger, Rwanda, Somalia, Sudan, Tanzania, and Zimbabwe. There have been great improvements in many of these countries and as of 2015 these are

the new estimates: Afghanistan is 396, Angola 447, Central African Republic 882, Chad 856, Ethiopia 353, Guinea-Bissau 549, Malawi 634, Mali 587, Niger 553, Rwanda 290, Somalia 732, Sudan, 311 (not including South Sudan, which is estimated between 789 and over 2,000 per 100,000 live births), Tanzania 398, and Zimbabwe 443, data.worldbank.org/indicator/SH.STA.MMRT.

9. Tina Rosenburg, "Reverse Foreign Aid," *New York Times*, March 25, 2007.

10. Retention of midwives, especially in rural areas, is a major challenge for many countries, one that threatens to negate all the hard work and resources invested in their training. Priya Shetty reports. "More midwives needed to improve maternal and newborn survival," *Bulletin of the World Health Organization*, 2013, unfpa.org/press/ world-needs-midwives-more-ever-keep-more-women-babies-alive-say-global-health-actors.

11. Wendy Graham, Achieving MDG 5: A Global Perspective, presentation given at the National Consultative Meeting on the Reduction of Maternal Mortality in Ghana: Partnership for Action, MOH, Ghana, October 2008.

12. Oona M.R. Campbell and Wendy J. Graham, on behalf of the *Lancet* Maternal Survival Series Steering Group, "Strategies for Reducing Maternal Mortality: Getting on with What Works," *Lancet* 368, no. 9543 (October 7, 2006): 1284–99.

13. Carine Ronsmans and Wendy J. Graham, on behalf of the *Lancet* Maternal Survival Series Steering Group, "Maternal Mortality: Who, When, Where, and Why," *Lancet* 368, no. 9542 (September 2006), doi.org/10.1016/S0140-6736(06)69380-X; Partnership for Maternal, Newborn and Child Health (website), World Health Organization, who.int/pmnch/en.

14. Information given in text on Sri Lanka and Uganda, found in United Kingdom, House of Commons, International Development Committee. *Maternal Health: Fifth Report of Session, 2007–2008*, vol. 1 (London: The Stationery Office, 2008), p. 17, publications. parliament.uk/pa/cm200708/cmselect/cmintdev/66/66i.pdf, 17; information on Ghana in Ibid., 18; information on Nepal in Ibid., 36.

15. Hon. Jim Abbott, *Hansard House of Commons Debates* 68 (June 4, 2009), who.int/pmnch/media/membernews/2009/200906_canadianresolution.pdf.
16. PMCH for maternal health requested and was refused $10.2 billion. See who.int/pmnch/media/mnchnews/2008/UNHLEonMDGs-mediaclips.pdf.
17. Toni Johnson, "Global Health Spending Priorities," *Council of Foreign Relations*, (October 6, 2008).
18. "Why Do So Many Women Still Die in Pregnancy or Childbirth?" World Health Organization, 2015, who.int/features/qa/12/en/index.html.
19. Ibid.
20. "Goal: Improve Maternal Health," Millennium Development Goals, UNICEF, unicef.org/mdg/maternal.html.
21. Richard Horton, "Maternal Mortality: Surprise, Hope, and Urgent Action," *Lancet*, 375, issue 9726 (May 8, 2010): 1581–82.
22. "Tackling Maternal Health 'Crisis,'" IRIN, November 30, 2011, irinnews.org/printreport.aspx?reportid=94352.
23. "Bush Administration Withholds UNFPA Funding for Seventh Year," Guttmacher Institute, June 27, 2008, guttmacher.org/media/inthenews/2008/06/27/index.html.
24. "WHO: Global Maternal Mortality Declines by More than One-Third," Voice of America News, September 14, 2010, voanews.com/english/news/health/WHO-Global-Maternal-Mortality-Declines-by-More-Than-One-Third-103009274.html.
25. National Bureau of Statistics (NBS) [Tanzania] and ICF Macro, *Tanzania Demographic and Health Survey 2010* (Dar es Salaam, Tanzania: NBS and ICF Macro, 2011), measuredhs.com/pubs/pdf/FR243/FR243[24June2011].pdf, 118.
26. The *2007 Demographic and Health Survey* suggests there is a "72 percent decline in child mortality and … 51 percent decline in under-five mortality." National Institute of Population Research and Training (NIPORT) and Macro International, *Bangladesh Demographic and Health Survey 2007* (Dhaka, Bangladesh and Calverton, MD: NIPORT, Mitra and Associates, and Macro

International, March 2009), p. 101, measuredhs.com/pubs/pdf/FR207/FR207[April-10-2009].pdf.

27. "Ghana is well on the way …" and "Table 4: Gender Inequality Index and related indicators," *Human Development Report, 2011*, pg. 141, hdr.undp.org/sites/default/files/reports/271/hdr_2011_en_complete.pdf.

28. Marcus Pistor, "Official Development Assistance Spending, in Brief," August 22, 2007, publications.gc.ca/collections/collection_2007/lop-bdp/eb/prb0710-e.pdf.

29. Campbell Clark, "G8 Pledges Fall Short of What's Needed," *Globe and Mail*, June 25, 2010. In the Muskoka initiative there was $5 billion in G8 pledges for maternal and child health. This is to be boosted by the $2.3 billion additional contributions from six G8 countries and the Gates Foundation. Canada pledged $1.1 billion. Canada's funding will focus on high-risk countries: Haiti, Afghanistan, Mali, Tanzania, and Mozambique.

30. For more information, see the Every Mother Counts website: everymothercounts.org.

31. For more information, visit UNICEF at unicef.org/corporate_partners/index_52225.html.

Chapter 8: We Are Still Waiting

1. Fistula survivors addressed the Deliver Now Conference held in the United Kingdom in 2007, and in Washington, D.C., in 2010, which focused attention on the poor progress addressing maternal health globally. Fistula survivors also addressed the U.S. Congress, mobilizing money from the United States for the Campaign to End Fistula, in a context when the Americans had stopped all money to the United Nations Population Fund.

2. Gretchen Roedde et al., *Bangladesh Country Report Evaluation of the Campaign to End Fistula* (Belgium: hera/New York: UNFPA, 2009).

3. Ibid.

4. Mihaela Minca, "Midwifery in Bangladesh: In-Depth Country Analysis" (background document prepared for UNFPA's *State of the*

World's Midwifery Report, 2011). The model for training these CS-BAs had originated in Indonesia, where the *bidan di desa*, received financial support from the community but were trained with government support. In Bangladesh they received additional training to deliver babies safely, paid for by government and managed technically by the Society of Obstetricians and Gynecologists, Bangladesh, with support from the United Nations Population Fund. They received their salaries from government for their work in family planning, prenatal, and child care but also received additional payment, such as a sari, from the women they delivered.

5. World Health Organization, *Health Financing Strategy for the Asia Pacific Region (2010–2015)* (Geneva, Switzerland: WHO Press, 2009), p. 27, wpro.who.int/publications/docs/Healthfinancingstrategy_6188.pdf?ua=1.

6. Ties J. Boerma et al., "Countdown to 2030: Tracking Progress Towards Universal Coverage for Reproductive, Maternal, Newborn and Child Health," *Lancet* 391, no. 10129 (January 2018).

7. Ibid.

8. National Population Commission (NPC) [Nigeria] and ICF International, *Nigeria Demographic and Health Survey 2013* (Abuja, Nigeria and Rockville, MD, USA: NPC and ICF International), dhsprogram.com/pubs/pdf/FR293/FR293.pdf.

ENDINGS

1. National Department of Health, *Ministerial Task Force on Maternal Health in Papua New Guinea* (Papua New Guinea: National Department of Health, 2009), p. 1, health.gov.pg/publications/Ministerial%20Taskforce%20Report.pdf.

2. The money seemed to have disappeared, lost in a political struggle between the Departments of Health and Planning. Some maternity wards were upgraded, but the bills were not paid, for example, at the Catholic Divine Word University in Madang. Most upgrades had been planned since 2006, with carefully done drawings, but could now not be financed.

3. There are different kinds of sing-sings when people gather, and feast, and dance and sing. Some might celebrate a marriage; some can be extremely dangerous, such as one that declares tribal war or a compensation sing-sing that arranges terms of settlement after a war.

4. Countdown to 2015, "Tanzania [country profile]," *Accountability for Maternal, Newborn and Child Survival — The 2013 Update* (Geneva, Switzerland: World Health Organization and UNICEF, 2013), who. int/woman_child_accountability/ierg/reports/Countdown_Account-ability_2013Report.pdf.

5. TDHS 2010.

6. Tanzania Country Study (Gretchen Roedde), "Formative Evaluation of Canada's Contribution to the Maternal, Newborn and Child Health (MNCH) Initiative," December 2015.

7. Ibid.

8. "Bhutan: WHO Statistical Profile," World Health Organization, last updated January 2015, who.int/gho/countries/btn.pdf?uaj=1. See also "Global Affairs Canada: Formative Evaluation of Canada's Contribution to the Maternal, Newborn and Child Health (MNCH) Initiative 2016. Nigeria Country Study (Gretchen Roedde), international. gc.ca/gac-amc/publications/evaluation/2016/eval_mnch-smne.aspx-?lang=eng. Nigeria Demographic and Health Survey 2013, dhspro-gram.com/pubs/pdf/FR293/FR293.pdf profiles.countdown2030. org/#/cp/NGA.

9. World Bank, *Country Partnership Strategy for the Kingdom of Bhutan for the Period of FY2015–19* (Washing, DC: World Bank group, 2014), documents.worldbank.org/curated/en/612871468205491416/pdf/885970CPS0P148000Box385310B00OUO090.pdf.

10. UNICEF, *UNICEF Annual Report 2013 – Bhutan* (2013), unicef.org/about/annualreport/files/Bhutan_COAR_2013.pdf.

11. Denise Darmawikarta, and Alexander Levit, "The Baby Blues: Challenges and Limitations of Delivering Obstetrics Care in Rural Canada," *University of Western Ontario Medical Journal* 83, no. 1 (2014), uwomj.com/wp-content/uploads/2014/10/v82no1_08.pdf.

APPENDIX 3

1. "Countdown to 2030: Tracking Progress Towards Universal Coverage for Reproductive, Maternal, Newborn, and Child Health," *Lancet*, January 30, 2018. DOI: doi.org/10.1016/S0140-6736(18)30104-1.
2. United Nations, Sustainable Development Goals, un.org/sustainabledevelopment.
3. Other tools to assess these indicators can be found at hdr.undp.org/en/media/hdr_2011_en_table4.pdf. Human Development Report 2011.

IMAGE CREDITS

Index

Page numbers in italics refer to photographs and their captions.

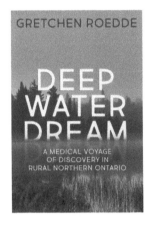

Deep Water Dream

A hopeful memoir that shares the author's voyage of discovery as a mother, wife, and physician in underserved communities in northern Ontario.

In underserved areas of Canada, the communities themselves can be one of the strongest parts of the health care team. Dr. Gretchen Roedde shows how local communities play a major role in responding to illness, birth, and death, making each more meaningful and bearable.

In *Deep Water Dream*, Roedde recounts stories from her long career — from working with a Cree community in developing a medical dictionary in their own language, to training community-based health workers, to delivering Amish babies in her own home. Roedde redraws the boundaries between physician and community, strengthening the capacity to care for those close by, and offers a hopeful and powerful example to the rest of the world.

Book Credits

Developmental Editor: Allison Hirst
Project Editor: Elena Radic
Copy Editor: Robyn So
Proofreader: Megan Beadle

Designer: Laura Boyle

Publicist: Elham Ali

Dundurn

Publisher: J. Kirk Howard
Vice-President: Carl A. Brand
Editorial Director: Kathryn Lane
Artistic Director: Laura Boyle
Production Manager: Rudi Garcia
Publicity Manager: Michelle Melski
Manager, Accounting and Technical Services: Livio Copetti

Editorial: Allison Hirst, Dominic Farrell, Jenny McWha, Rachel Spence,
Elena Radic, Melissa Kawaguchi
Marketing and Publicity: Kendra Martin, Elham Ali,
Tabassum Siddiqui, Heather McLeod
Design and Production: Sophie Paas-Lang

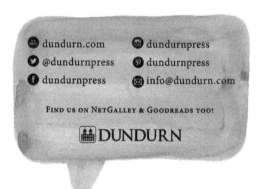

dundurn.com   dundurnpress
@dundurnpress   dundurnpress
dundurnpress   info@dundurn.com

FIND US ON NETGALLEY & GOODREADS TOO!

DUNDURN